OBSTETRICS AND GYNECOLOGY ADVANCES

ROBOTIC GYNECOLOGY

FROM CONCEPT TO APPLICATIONS

Obstetrics and Gynecology Advances

Additional books in this series can be found on Nova's website under the Series tab.

Additional e-books in this series can be found on Nova's website under the e-book tab.

OBSTETRICS AND GYNECOLOGY ADVANCES

ROBOTIC GYNECOLOGY

FROM CONCEPT TO APPLICATIONS

CHRISTOS R. IAVAZZO, M.D., PH.D.
AND
IOANNIS D. GKEGKES, M.D.

NOVA BIOMEDICAL

New York

For permission to use material from this book please contact us:
Telephone 631-231-7269; Fax 631-231-8175
Web Site: http://www.novapublishers.com

Library of Congress Cataloging-in-Publication Data

ISBN: 978-1-63321-813-0

Library of Congress Control Number: 2014948043

Published by Nova Science Publishers, Inc. † New York

Contents

Introduction

Ιθάκη

ΣαβγειςστονπηγαιμόγιατηνΙθάκη,
να εύχεσαι νάναι μακρύς ο δρόμος,
γεμάτος περιπέτειες, γεμάτος γνώσεις.
Τους Λαιστρυγόνας και τους Κύκλωπας,
τον θυμωμένο Ποσειδώνα μη φοβάσαι,
τέτοια στον δρόμο σου ποτέ σου δεν θα βρεις,
αν μέν' η σκέψις σου υψηλή, αν εκλεκτή
συγκίνησις το πνεύμα και το σώμα σου αγγίζει.
Τους Λαιστρυγόνας και τους Κύκλωπας,
τον άγριο Ποσειδώνα δεν θα συναντήσεις,
αν δεν τους κουβανείς μες στην ψυχή σου,
αν η ψυχή σου δεν τους στήνει εμπρός σου.

Να εύχεσαι νάναι μακρύς ο δρόμος.
Πολλά τα καλοκαιρινά πρωιά να είναι
που με τι ευχαρίστησι, με τι χαρά
θα μπαίνεις σε λιμένας πρωτοειδωμένους·
να σταματήσεις σ' εμπορεία Φοινικικά,
και τες καλές πραγμάτειες ν' αποκτήσεις,
σεντέφια και κοράλλια, κεχριμπάρια κ' έβενους,
και ηδονικά μυρωδικά κάθε λογής,
όσο μπορείς πιο άφθονα ηδονικά μυρωδικά·
σε πόλεις Αιγυπτιακές πολλές να πας,
να μάθεις και να μάθεις απ' τους σπουδασμένους.

Πάντα στον νου σου νάχεις την Ιθάκη.
Το φθάσιμον εκεί είν' ο προορισμός σου.
Αλλά μη βιάζεις το ταξείδι διόλου.
Καλλίτερα χρόνια πολλά να διαρκέσει·
και γέρος πια ν' αράξεις στο νησί,
πλούσιος με όσα κέρδισες στον δρόμο,
μη προσδοκώντας πλούτη να σε δώσει η Ιθάκη.

Η Ιθάκη σ' έδωσε τ' ωραίο ταξείδι.
Χωρίς αυτήν δεν θάβγαινες στον δρόμο.
Άλλα δεν έχει να σε δώσει πια.

Κι αν πτωχική την βρεις, η Ιθάκη δεν σε γέλασε.
Έτσι σοφός που έγινες, με τόση πείρα,
ήδη θα το κατάλαβες η Ιθάκες τι σημαίνουν.

(Κ.Π. Καβάφη, Από τα Ποιήματα 1897-1933, Ίκαρος 1984)

Ithaka

As you set out for Ithaka
hope the voyage is a long one,
full of adventure, full of discovery.
Laistrygonians and Cyclops,
angry Poseidon—don't be afraid of them:
you'll never find things like that on your way
as long as you keep your thoughts raised high,
as long as a rare excitement
stirs your spirit and your body.
Laistrygonians and Cyclops,
wild Poseidon—you won't encounter them
unless you bring them along inside your soul,
unless your soul sets them up in front of you.

Hope the voyage is a long one.
May there be many a summer morning when,
with what pleasure, what joy,
you come into harbors seen for the first time;
may you stop at Phoenician trading stations
to buy fine things,
mother of pearl and coral, amber and ebony,
sensual perfume of every kind—
as many sensual perfumes as you can;
and may you visit many Egyptian cities
to gather stores of knowledge from their scholars.
Keep Ithaka always in your mind.
Arriving there is what you are destined for.
But do not hurry the journey at all.
Better if it lasts for years,
so you are old by the time you reach the island,
wealthy with all you have gained on the way,
not expecting Ithaka to make you rich.

Ithaka gave you the marvelous journey.
Without her you would not have set out.
She has nothing left to give you now.

And if you find her poor, Ithaka won't have fooled you.
Wise as you will have become, so full of experience,
you will have understood by then what these Ithakas mean.

(C.P. Cavafis, Collected Poems. Translated by Edmund Keeley and Philip Sherrard. Edited by George Savidis. Revised Edition. Princeton University Press, 1992)

Preface

This book entitled "Robotic Gynaecology: From Concept to Applications" serves to provide a comprehensive, evidence based and updated review on the role of Da Vinci® robot in gynaecological operations. All of the chapters have been organized with a critical eye to the needs of the modern minimal access gynaecologist. This handbook is written in an easy-to-read format. Indications, patient preparation, role of the team members, operative techniques, and strategies for avoiding and managing complications are included for the complete spectrumin robotic gynaecology. It also places special focus on tips and management of pitfalls. The book also includes a good number of tables and images which make it informative and educational.

Dr Iavazzo would like to thank his wife Fotinie for standing beside him throughout his career and writing this book. She has been his inspiration and motivation for continuing to improve his knowledge and move his career forward. He dedicates this book to her. He would like to thank his parents and sister for their support and patience during his ''journey'' to follow his professional ambitions. Last but not least, he would like to thank his mentors, Mr Simon Butler-Manuel and Mr Anil Tailor, world known experts in Robotic Gynaecology who gave him the opportunity to be trained by the best for over a year in Royal Surrey County Hospital, Guildford, United Kingdom.

Dr Gkegkes would like to thank his teachers, his parents and sister and to all who believed and support his effort to be better person and scientist.

We would really like to thank Nadya Gotsiridze-Columbus, President of Nova Science Publishers, Inc. for providing us with the opportunity to become the lead authors for this book. We appreciate that she believed in us to provide the leadership and knowledge to make this book a reality.

We hope that this manual is going to find a home in the pocket, locker or briefcase of all gynaecologists interested in robotic surgery and be a valuable resource for a broad spectrum of clinicians, healthcare professionals and students. We believe that the information contained in this book will enhance the skills of the surgeon in order to offer excellent preoperative, intraoperative and postoperative care.

Christos Iavazzo, M.D., MSc, Ph.D.
Gynaecological Oncology Department,
Christie Hospital, Manchester, United Kingdom

Ioannis D. Gkegkes, M.D.
First Department of Surgery,
General Hospital of Attica "KAT", Athens, Greece

Chapter 1

Evolution of Robots throughout History

A lot of descriptions of androids mimicking robots could be found in mythology and history. For example:

- The statue of Memnon – King of Ethiopia, which was created by Amenhotepin ancient Egypt, and was activating by the rising sun and playing music.

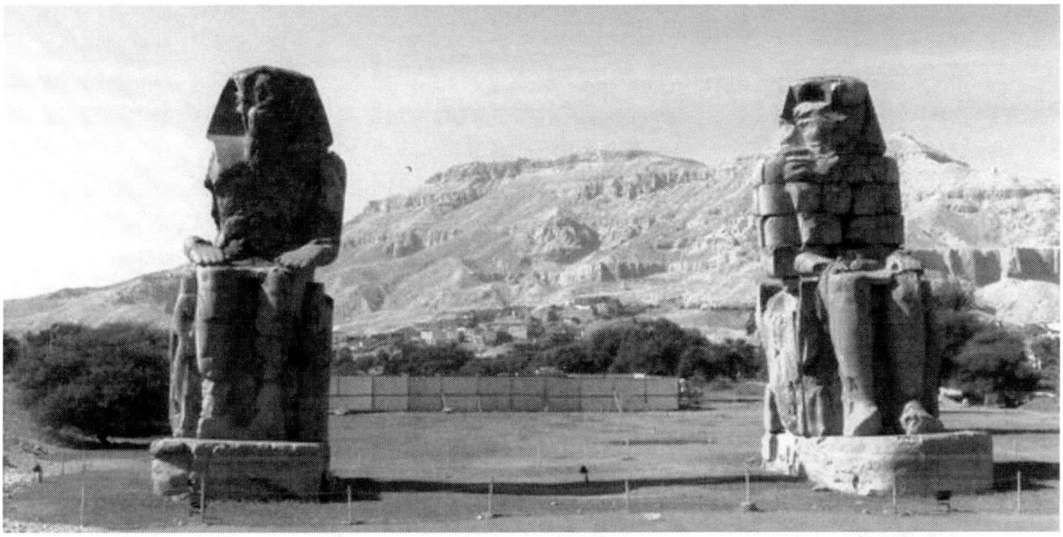

The statue of Memnon.

- In Greek mythology, Talos was another mechanical creature. According to the myth, Talos was a metallic giant made by copper, which was given by god Hephaestus at Minos, the king of Crete. The mission of Talos was to protect the island from enemies. The weak point of Talos was an artery which ran from his neck to his heel.

During the campaign of the Argonauts on the island of Crete, Talos was immobilized by Medea with the use of magic tricks and killed by her by cutting his artery.

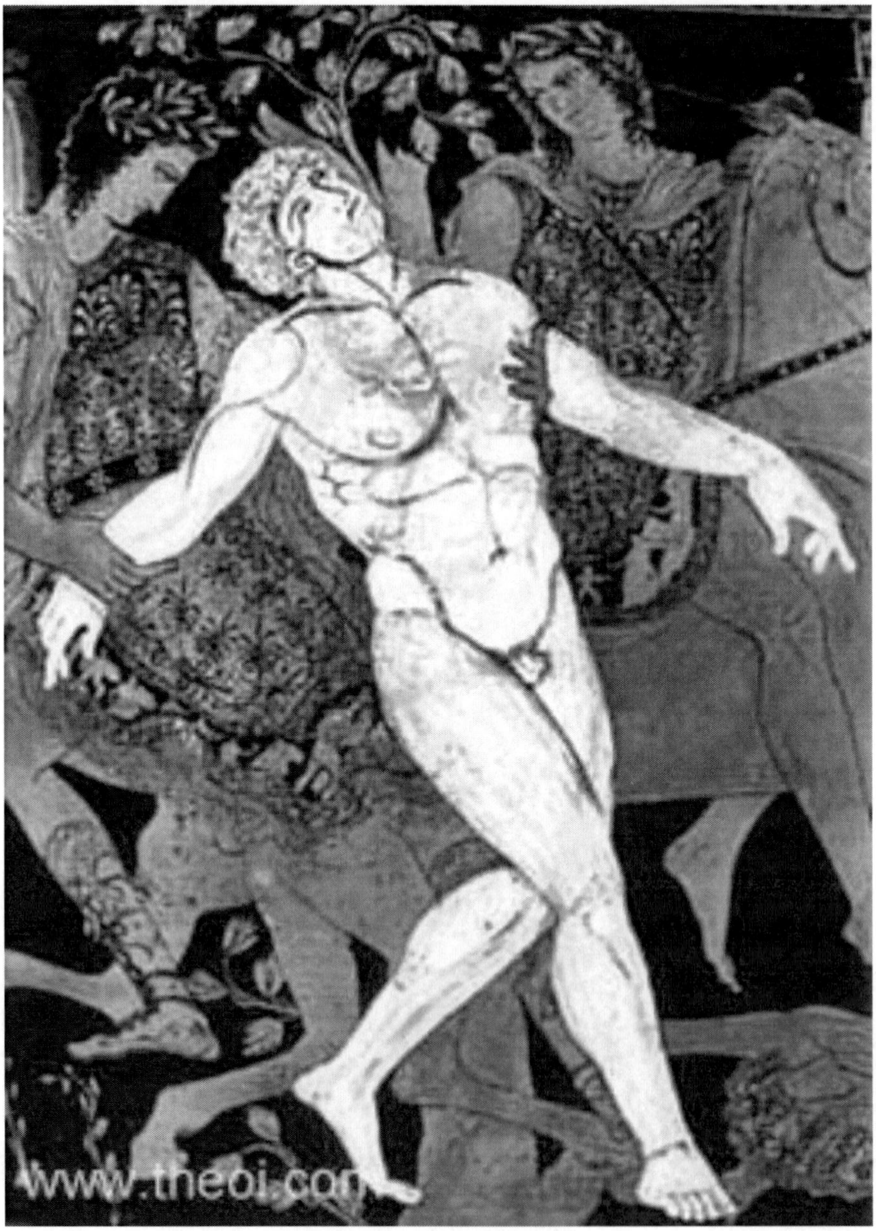

The death of Talos.

- In ancient China, emperor Yang (569-618 A.D.) of the Sui Dynasty requested from his engineers to create a wooden man which was mounted with a machine in its torso. Such a mechanism enabled it to stand up, sit down and worship on bended knees mimicking the movements of a servant.

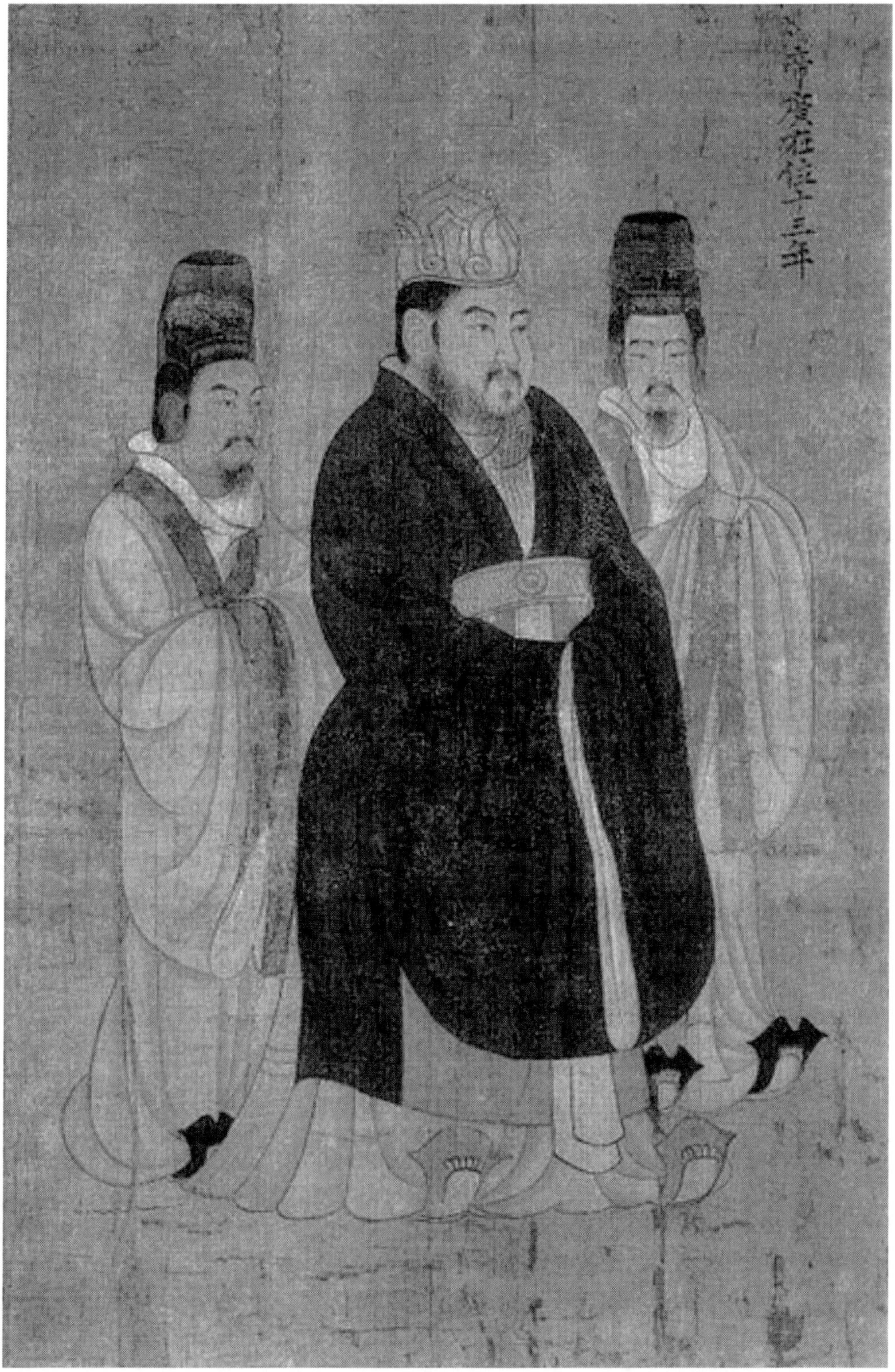

Emperor Yang.

- In the Arab world, Al-Jazari (1136-1206 A.C.), an Arab engineer, created a musical automaton, which was a boat with four automatic musicians that floated on a lake to entertain guests at royal gatherings.

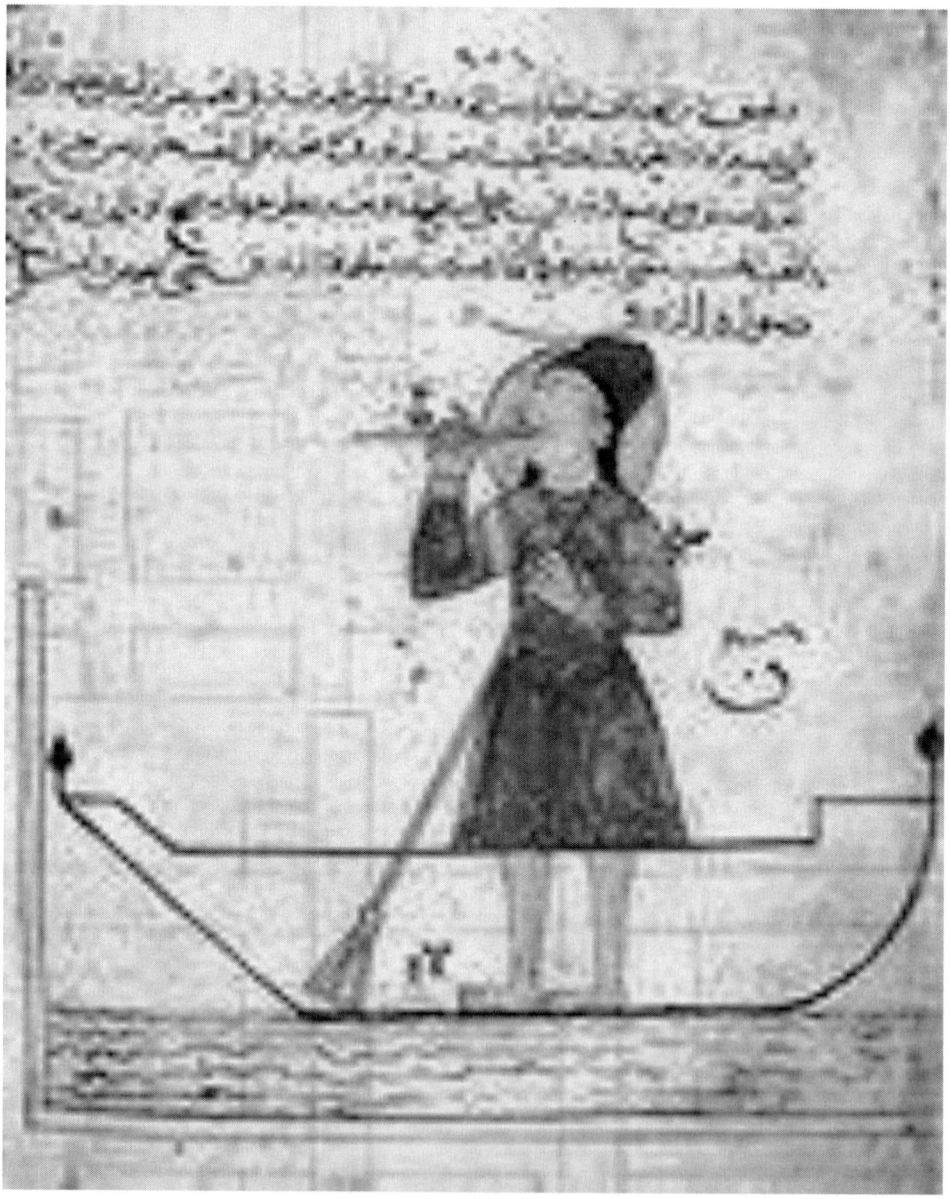

Musical automaton.

- Leonardo Da Vinci (1452-1519 A.C.) in the Renaissance, designed various machines, as the improvement of technical projects and the expansion of scientific studies in various fields including flying machines, reminiscent of gliders, helicopters and parachutes. Among other machines, Da Vinci built humanoid-robot which was used in medieval armor and was capable to make several human-like movements. Leonardo showed his automaton at the court of Milan, in 1495.

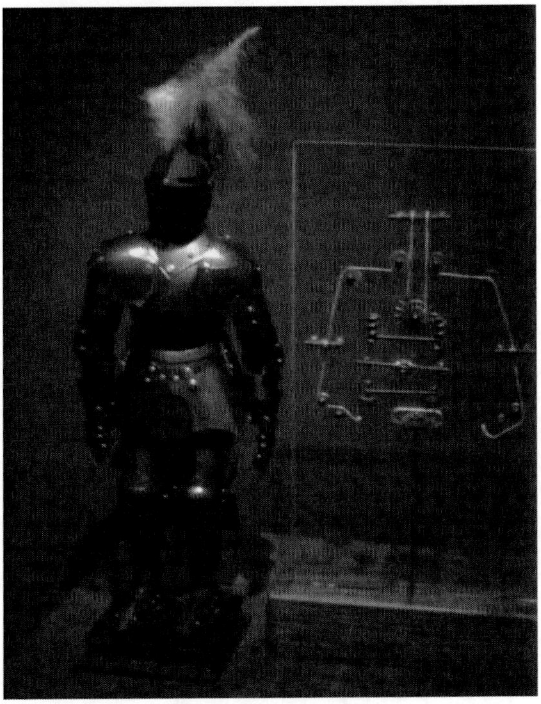

Da Vinci's knight.

- Czech writer Karel Capek (1890-1938 A.C.) was the first to use the term "robot" in his play "Rossum's Universal Robots", in 1923. In his play, robots are presented as small artificial anthropomorphic creatures which obey strictly to the commands of their master. At the end of the play, robots rebelled against their creators.

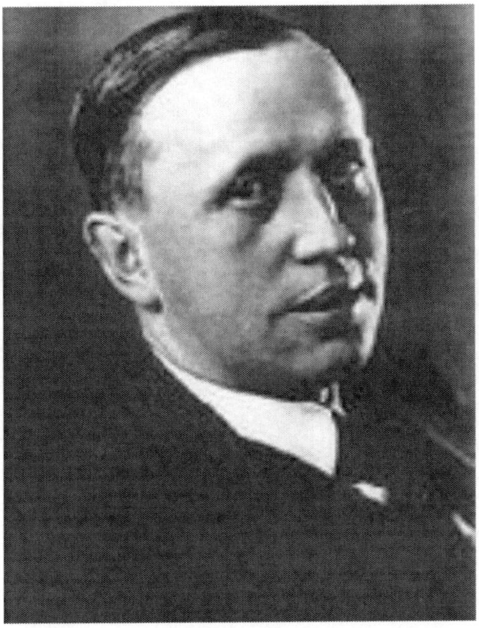

Karel Capek.

- In the 20th century, robots were used in the exploration of the oceans and of the space.
- Medical robots: The utilisation of robots in medicine began with the PUMA robot.

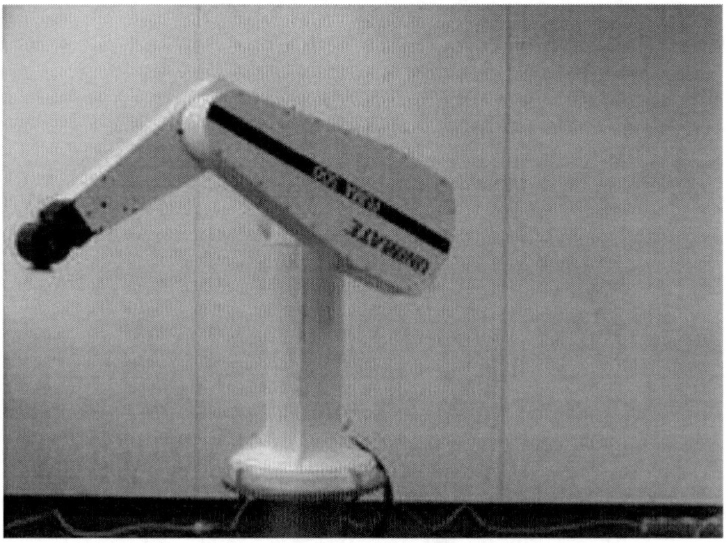

PUMA robot.

PUMA 560 was the robot used in brain biopsies in 1985, while the PROBOT robot in 1988 was applied in prostate surgery. In 1994, FDA approved the first surgical robot, called Aesop, with a single robotic arm which controlled the camera, allowing the surgeon to use both hands while operating. Two additional arms were added and in 1999, and the surgical system Zeus (Computer Motion) was created.

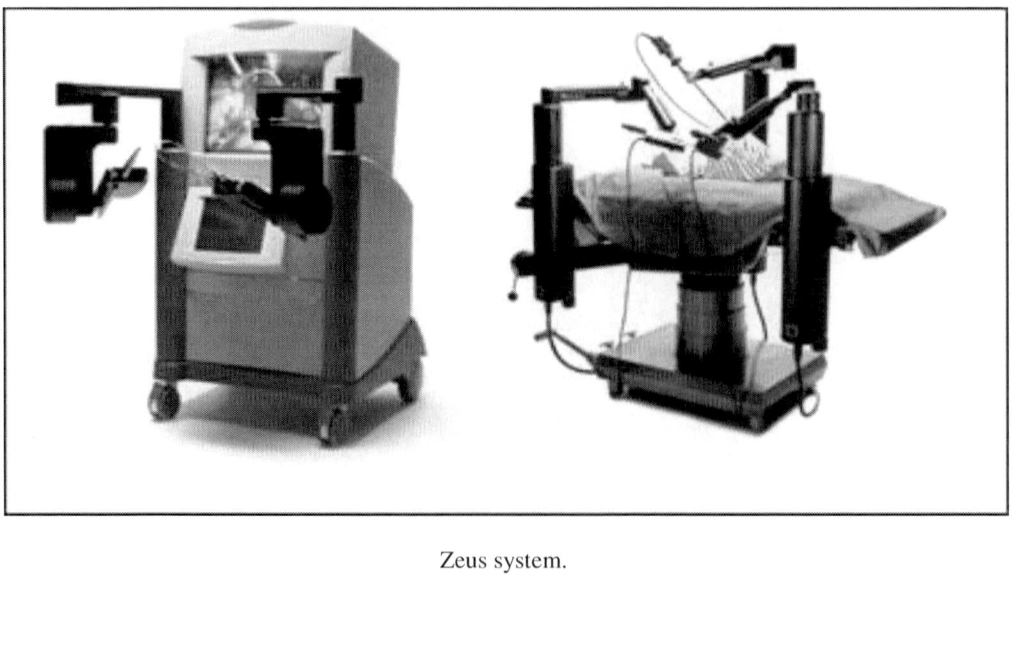

Zeus system.

The surgeon was situated at the control console and manipulated the surgical robotic tools. The surgical system Zeus, was used for the first telesurgery operative treatment in 2001, when surgeons in New York successfully completed a cholecystectomy in Strasbourg, France. In 1999, the Da Vinci robot (Intuitive Surgical Company) was the first to be used for a robotic-assisted surgery aortocoronary bypass.

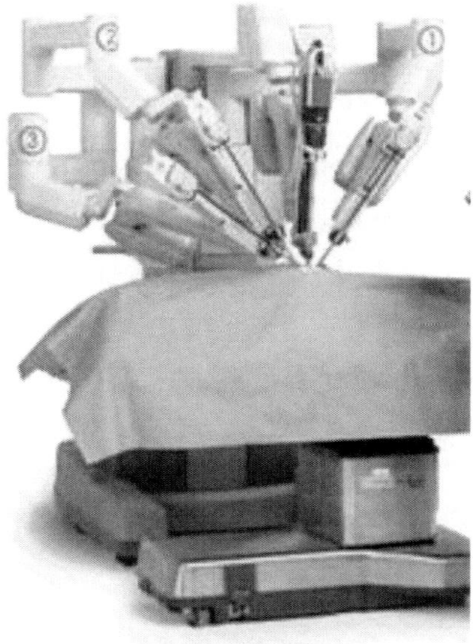

Da Vinci robot.

Computer Motion and Intuitive Surgical companies announced their merger in 2003. The era of robotic assisted surgery had begun.

Chapter 2

The Da Vinci Robot

The Da Vinci Robot is including the following parts which are necessary for its optimal use:

a) Master surgeon's console:

The surgeon uses the master console as an interface to operate the da Vinci surgical system. The console interprets the surgeon's body movements as input signals directed to the surgical cart. It also provides visual and force feedback to the surgeon.

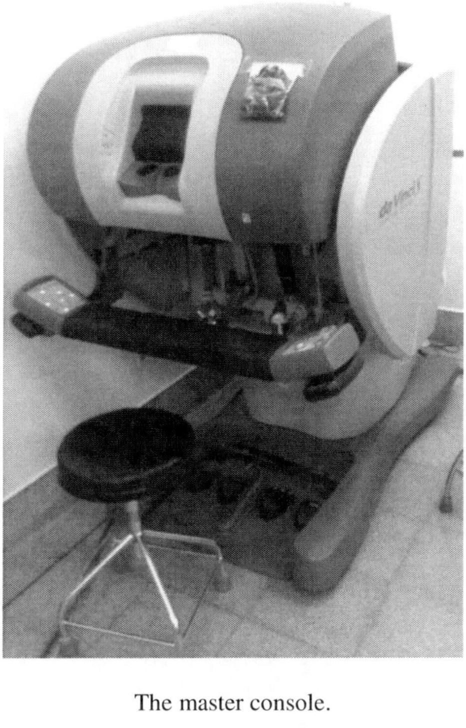

The master console.

The major components of the master surgeon's console include the connection, the stereoscopic viewer, the dual master controls, the foot pedals, and the control panels.

i) Connection:

The master surgeon's console is connected to the surgical cart via electric cables. It can be placed up to thirty feet away from the operating table.

ii) Stereoscopic Viewer:

Located at the console, the stereoscopic viewer provides visual feedback to the surgeon. It consists of two, separate, medical grade cathode ray tubes, one for each eye. The stereoscopic viewer presents the surgeon with a ten-fold magnified and three-dimensional image of the operative field, obtained by the dual channel endoscope at the surgical cart. The surgeon views the image by placing his or her head into the padded viewer, which contains sensors that detect the surgeon's head position. The robot arms are only activated when the surgeon is viewing.

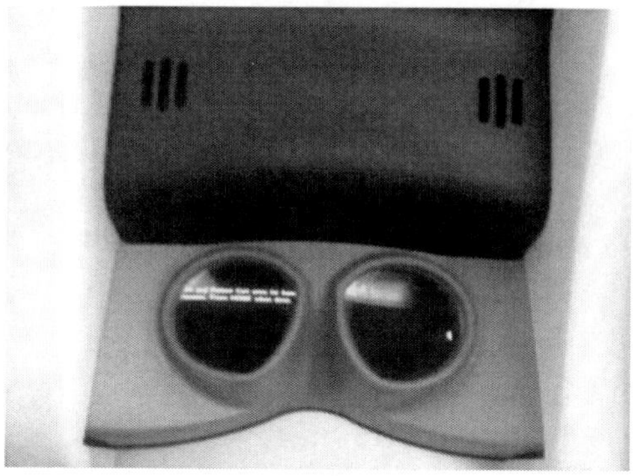

The stereoscopic viewer.

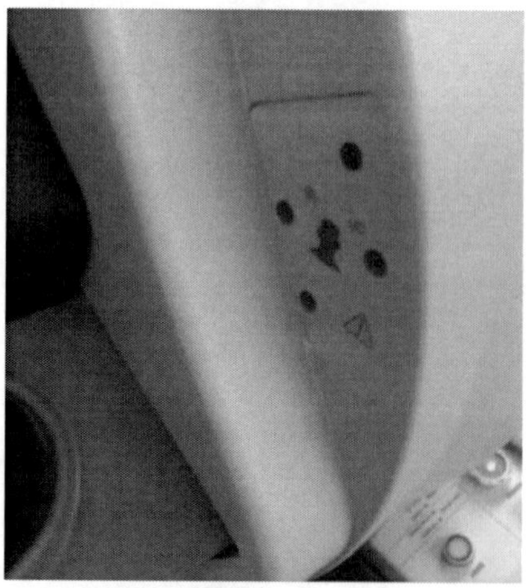

Sensors of head position.

iii) Dual master controls:

The dual master controls translate the surgeon's hand movements to the operation being performed on the patient with the surgical robotic arms. These controls are joystick-like devices patterned after Castro-style needle drivers, designed to provide the intuitiveness of operating with conventional surgical tools. The surgeon uses the controls by placing his or her fingers onto the master grips. These grips allow various types of movements including rotating, squeezing and sliding. The hand movements of the surgeon are directly translated into corresponding movements of the articulating instruments on the surgical robot arm. For example, squeezing together the levers of an individual master grip enables the surgeon to close the tips of a corresponding needle driver or forceps. There are also unique wristed instruments on the surgical robot arm that move according to the wrist movements of the surgeon. The master controls also provide the surgeon with gross force feedback.

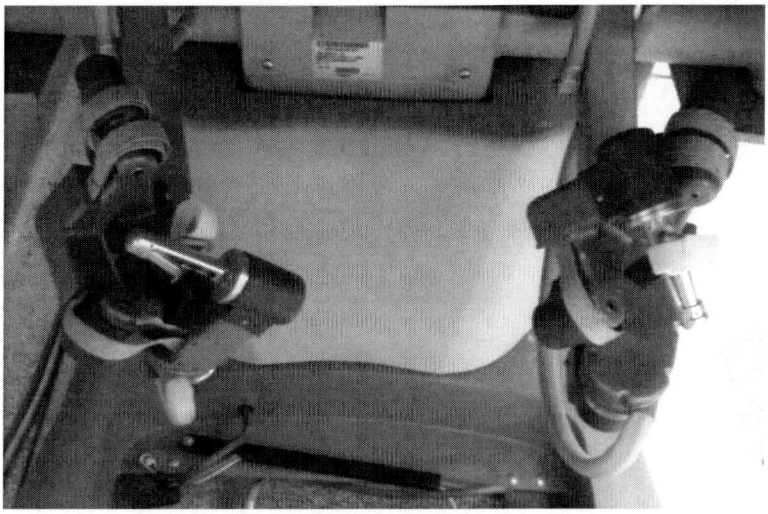

Master controls.

iv) Foot pedals:

The foot pedals on the master surgeon's console have various functions. The camera control pedal is used to manipulate the endoscope at the surgical cart. When the camera control pedal is depressed and held down, the master grips of the dual master controls are disengaged from the instruments. Instead, the surgeon has control over the movement of the endoscope. The clutch pedal allows the surgeon to disengage the master grips from the surgical cart, in order to reposition them into a more comfortable configuration without disturbing the instruments or the endoscope. The other camera pedals enable the surgeon to control camera focus and activate electrocautery.

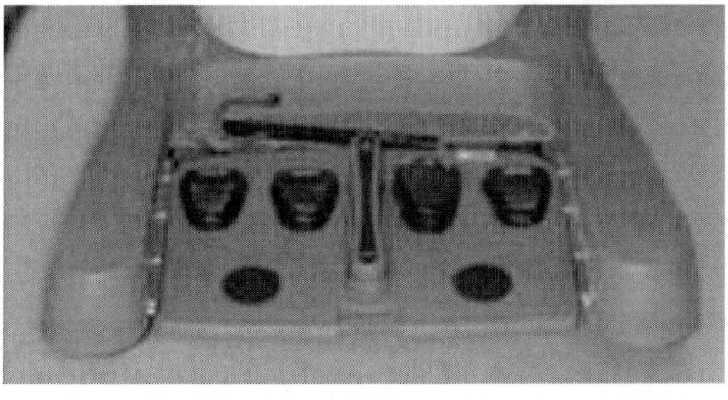

Foot pedals.

v) Control panels (user interface panel and user switch panel):

The control panels are used by the surgeon to calibrate the Da Vinci surgical system. They enable the surgeon to:

- Choose and calibrate either the 30 degree or 0 degree endoscope
- Adjust motion scaling
- Select camera angle (up or down)
- Change between three-dimensional and two-dimensional viewing
- Pace the system on and off standby
- Completely disengage the system

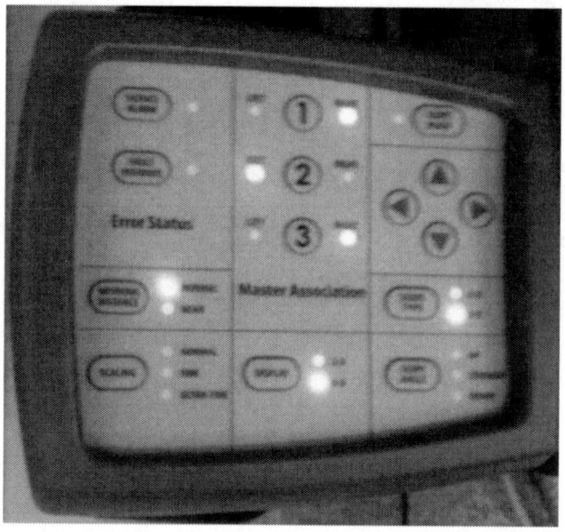

Left control panel.

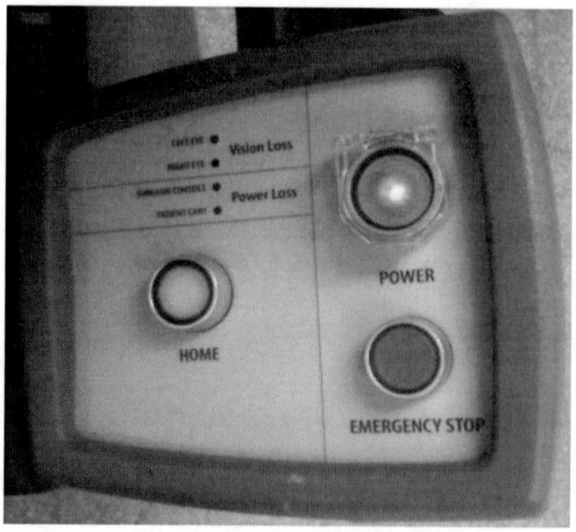

Right control panel.

b) Surgical cart:

The surgical cart is the robotic system at the patient's side that carries out the actual surgery for the surgeon. It is the "slave" component in the Da Vinci surgical system which means that all of its actions are the results of the input from the master surgeon's console.

During the surgery, the surgical cart is positioned adjacent to the operating table. Its position varies depending on the particular operation being performed. The major components of the surgical cart include three robotic operating arms, their articulating instruments, and the camera arm.

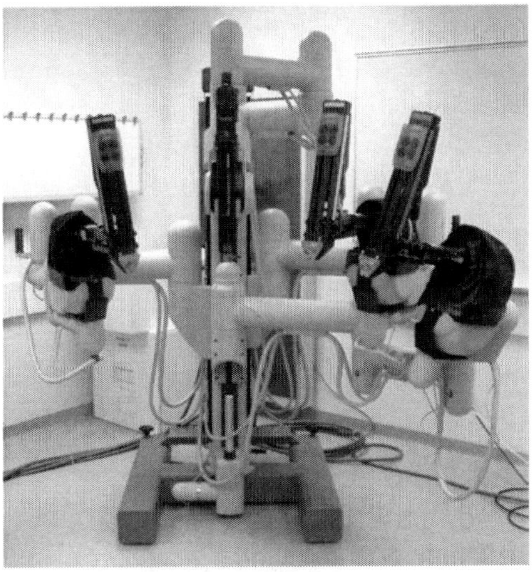

Surgical cart.

i) Robotic operating arms:

The robotic operating arms carry out operations guided by the surgeon from the master surgeon's console. These operating arms correspond to the left and right hand of the surgeon. They are motor-driven, cable-actuated, and mounted on a movable chassis. There are setup joint buttons that set up and position the robot arms. They allow for the arm's gross movements. To assist the operating surgeon, during a procedure, a patient-side assistant also has the option to use the clutch buttons to precisely move the robotic arms. The robotic arms move around a remote center determined by the setup joint position. They provide very steady fulcrum points for the instruments and trocars to move around – a big advantage over traditional laparoscopic surgery.

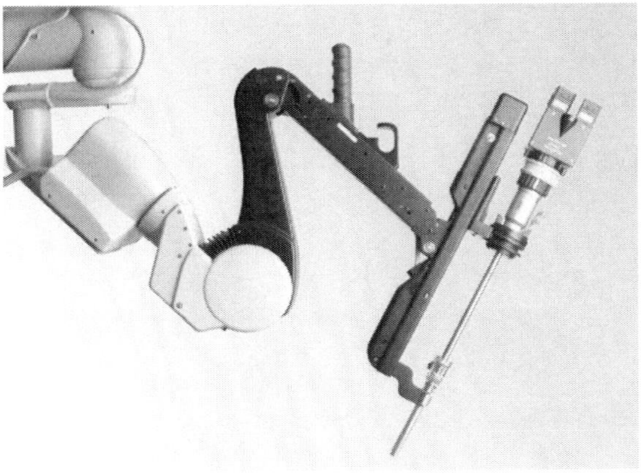

Operating arm.

ii) Articulating instruments:

The articulating instruments are the surgical tools available to the surgeon to carry out the operation. The articulating instruments are mounted onto the operating arms through unique sterile adaptors, which serve both as electrical and mechanical interfaces between the instruments and the robotic arms. These reusable adapters feature four notched wheels that match the corresponding wheels on the instruments. The mechanical forces are transmitted through these wheels, enabling the instruments' unique wristed movements and grip. Inside the articulating instruments, a series of tungsten cables are attached to the notched wheels, further transmitting the mechanical forces to the tips of the instruments. Furthermore, each instrument contains a microchip, which tells the robotic arm which particular instrument is being used and records the usage count. The Da Vinci system currently features 18 different surgical instrument tip configurations: including a variety of fully articulating graspers, forceps, blades, and needle drivers. The instruments utilized by the surgical system also include a number of energy-delivering instruments, such as a mono-polar hook, spatula cautery, bipolar forceps, and ultrasonic forceps. The Da Vinci instruments can be sterilized and, depending on the instrument, are reusable for up to 10-15 operations.

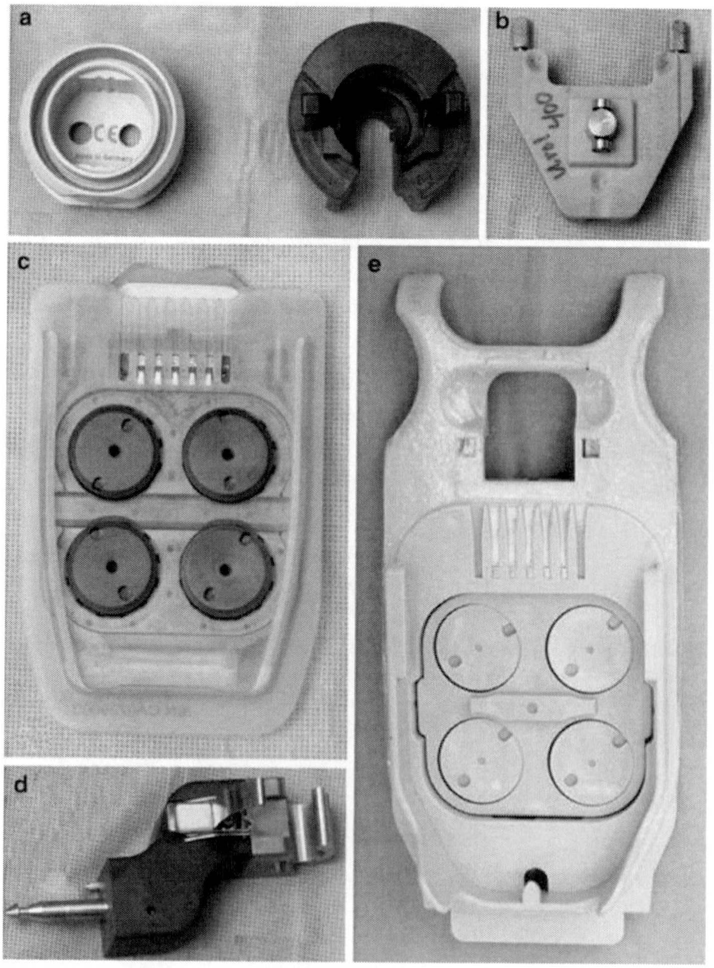

Articulating instruments (Continued).

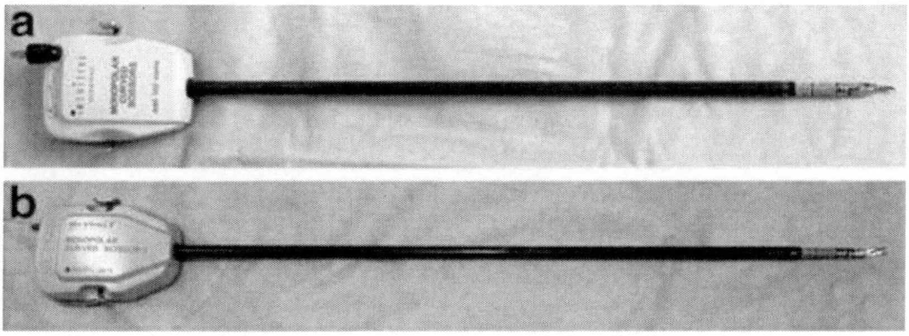

Articulating instruments.

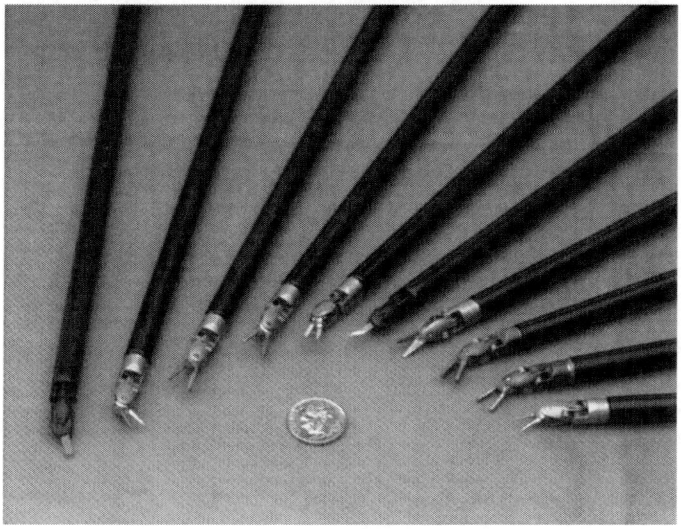

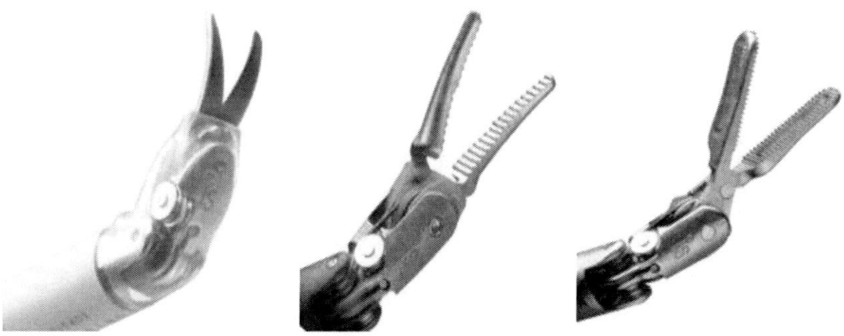

DaVinci instruments.

ii) Camera arm:

The camera arm is the mounting basis for the dual channel endoscope. It allows the surgeon to change, move, zoom and rotate his or her vision from the master surgeon's console. The dual channel endoscope mounted on the camera arm is attached to two separate, three-chip cameras. These cameras are further connected to the two separate camera control units on the vision cart. The endoscope is currently 12 mm in diameter and houses two separate 5 mm telescopes. It is available in 0 degree and 30 degree versions. The most commonly used configuration utilizes a wide-angle camera that provides a magnified 60 degree field of view. A higher magnification camera, with a narrower field of view, is also available.

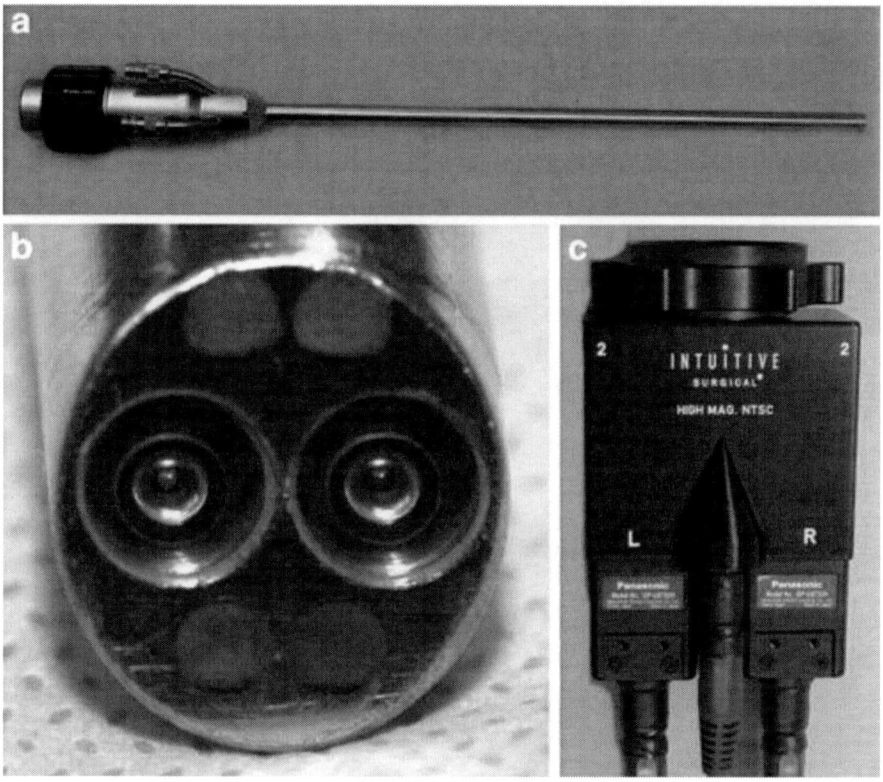

The endoscope.

iii) The fourth arm:

For additional purchase, a fourth arm is available for the Da Vinci surgical system. This extra operating arm can mount a third set of surgical instruments, in addition to the ones on the original two arms. This optional arm enables the surgeon to perform additional tasks such as applying counter traction and following running sutures. Only two of the three operating arms are controlled by the surgeon at the same time, and the switching between arms is made easy through the foot pedals.

c) Vision cart:

The vision cart of the Da Vinci surgical system is a simple movable tower that houses the dual light sources and camera control equipment. Typically, it also houses:

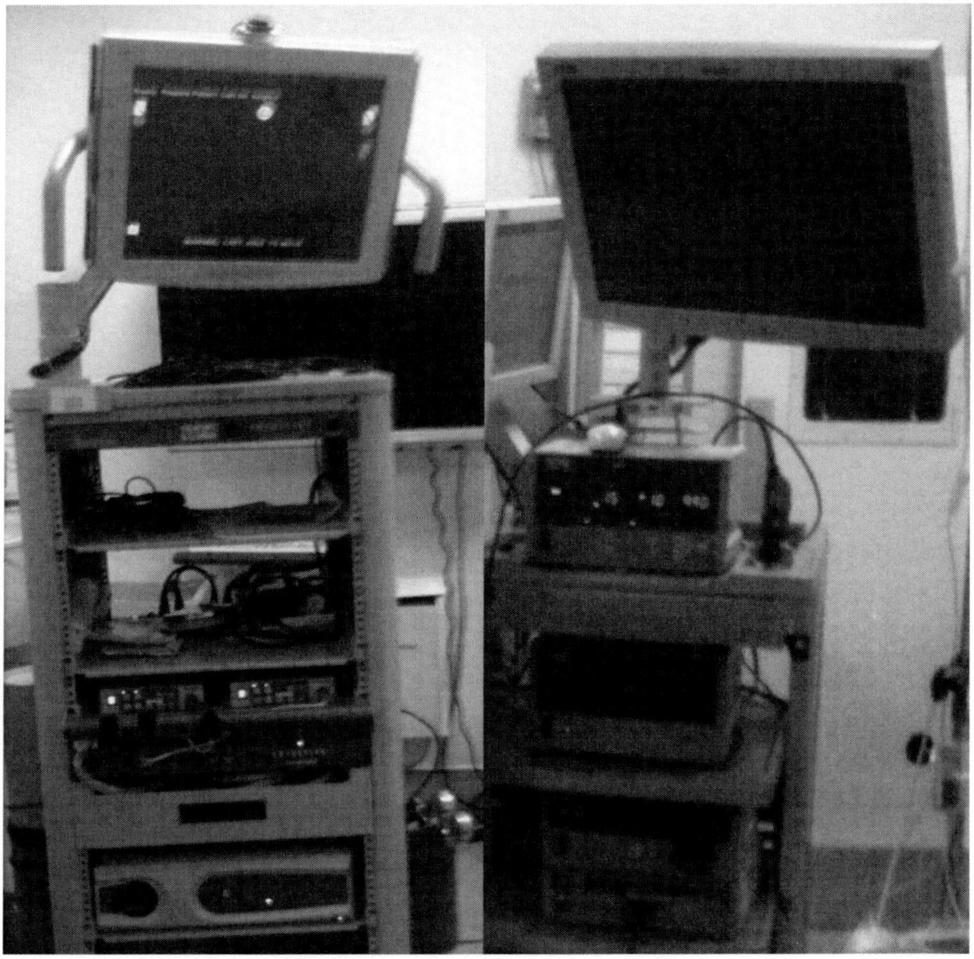

Vision cart.

i. An insufflation device
ii. A standard laparoscopic monitor for use by the patient-side assistant
iii. The imaging processing equipment necessary to process the camera signals that render the three-dimensional vision at the surgeon's console.

Chapter 3

Surgical Room, Positioning, Port Placement and Docking

The surgical room setting should be characterised by:

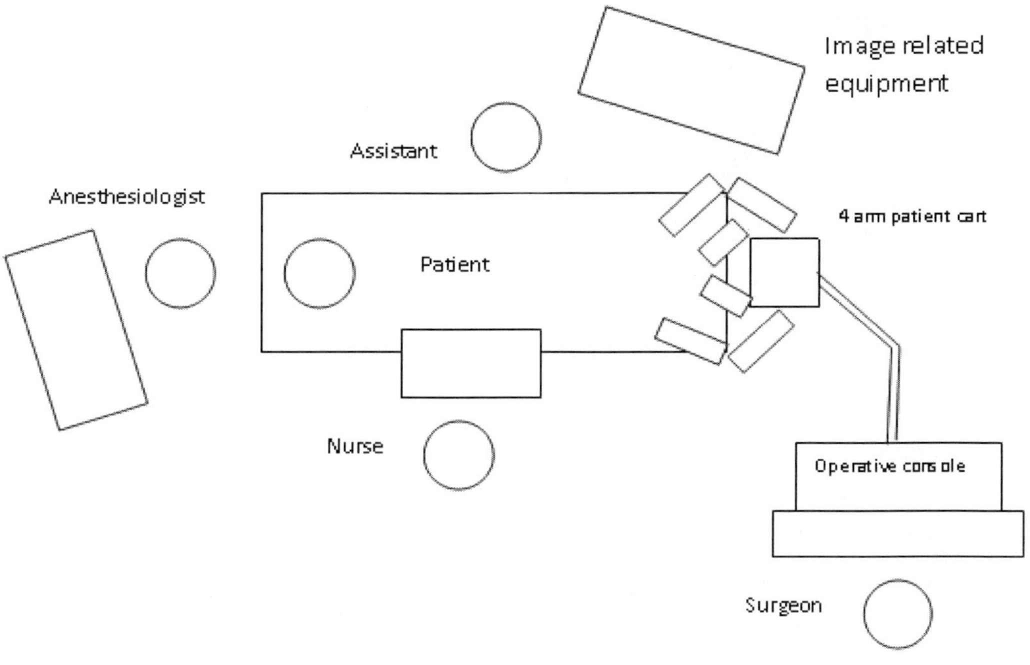

Surgical room setting.

Surgical room setting

- space for all the robotic components
- tension-free cable connections
- clear pathways for personnel to move freely around the room
- laparoscopic towers to hold the insufflator

- insufflation tank
- electrosurgical units
- video system
- extra monitors
- DVD recorder

The room should offer clear view of the patient from the surgeon console, as well as possibility of docking from several different angles.

Patient Positioning

The patient is positioned in modified lithotomy position with legs on Allen stirrups.

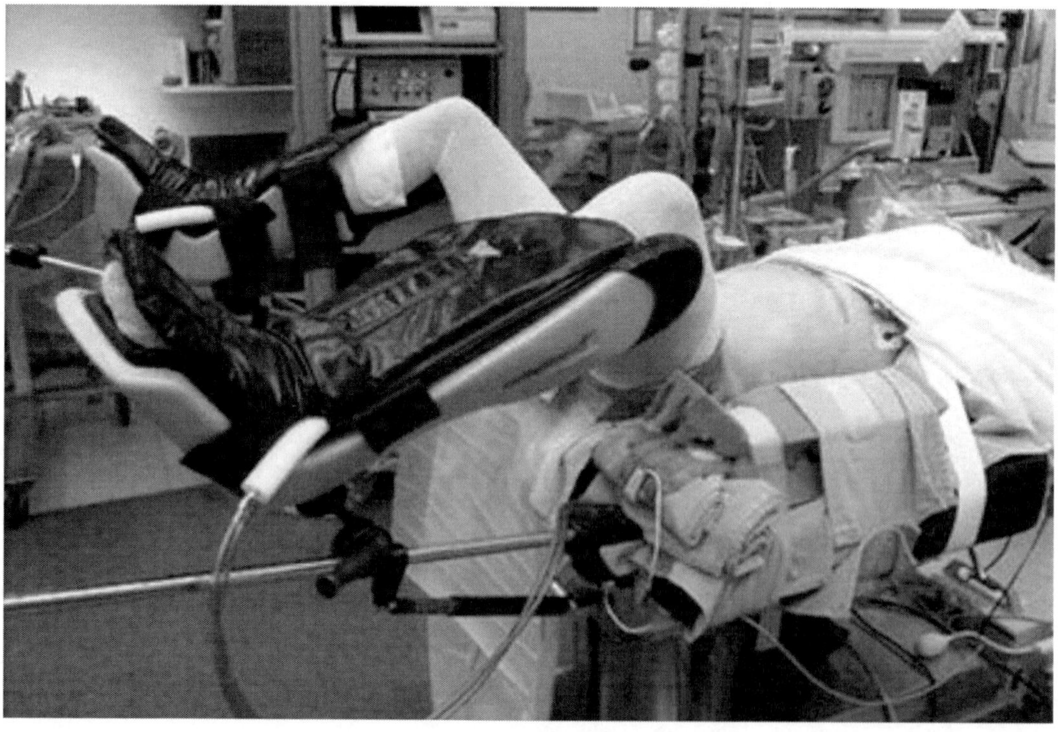

Patient positioning.

Patient is positioned on a gel pad to avoid sliding during Trendelenburg. The correct Trendelenburg position is checked with the use of a simple nautical inclinometer to identify the correct incline of the bed rapidly and precisely (28-30 degrees angle of incline). This application could easily be found even in smart phones.

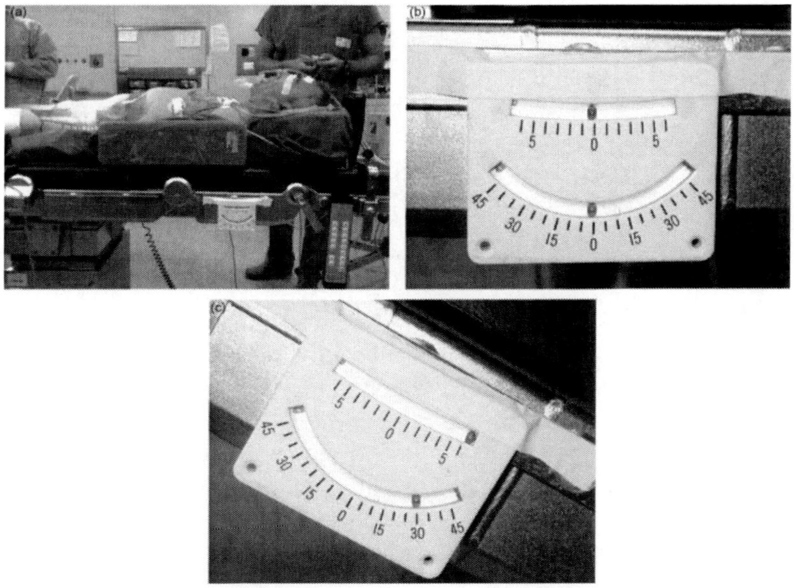

Inclinometer.

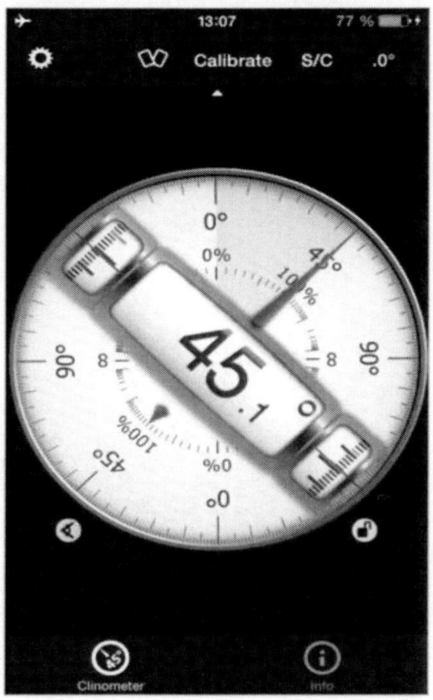

Inclinometer (smart phone application).

The patient's face and endotracheal tube are secured to avoid accidents during movement of the robotic endoscope. The arms are padded and positioned along side on arm boards. Thromboembolic stockings and sequential compression devices are used to prevent thromboembolic episodes. An upper body Bair Hugger is used above the xiphoid and insulated with a blanket. Surgical preparation is essential from the xiphoid to perineum to midaxillary lines.

Port Placement

The 12-mm primary trocar for the camera is placed in the umbilicus or above it in a way that the distance of the uterine fundus from the umbilical port is 10 cm. Once the abdomen is insufflated, the following landmarks are identified: the upper margin of the pubis bone, the anterosuperior iliac spine, bilaterally and a point on the midline at a distance of 15 cm from the pubis bone. The correct placement of the ports is crucial to avoid robotic arms collision. The operative trocars should be positioned bilaterally. More specifically, eight-millimeter lateral trocars are placed 8 to 10 cm laterally for the 2 robotic arms. In cases of bilateral pelvic lymph node dissection the trocars are placed more laterally to have adequate space.

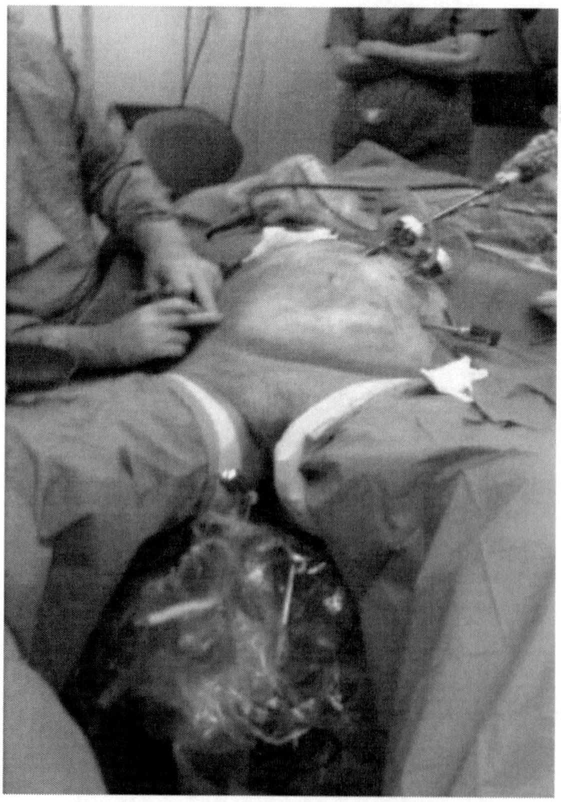

Port placement.

The trocar for the third robotic arm is placed on the right upper quadrant. An accessory 12-mm trocar is placed in the left upper quadrant for assistance. More analytically, the robotic arms on the right are placed at least 8 to 10 cm apart, with the lower port slightly above the anterior superior iliac spine and the upper port triangulated between the umbilical port and the lower port. The left-sided port is then placed roughly parallel to the lower right-sided port. An assistant's port is then placed cephalad and to the left of the umbilical trocar.

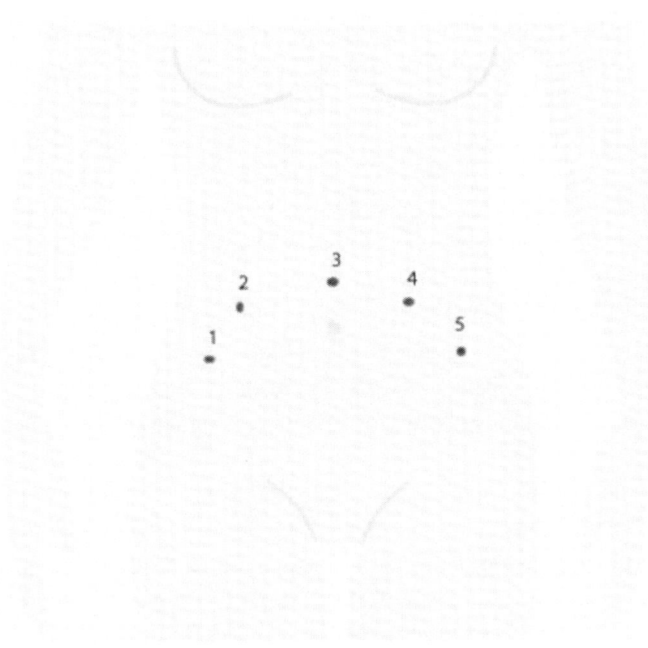

Correct port placement.

Docking

One member of the surgical team drives the patient cart while the surgeon guides the driver by using anatomic or room references. The nurse is driving the robot to the surgical table. To operate the motor drive, he/she unlocks the brakes and turns the shift switches on the base of the cart to the drive position and turns the throttle forward or backwards with the right hand. To move the cart without the motor drive assist, the nurse turns the shift switches to neutral.

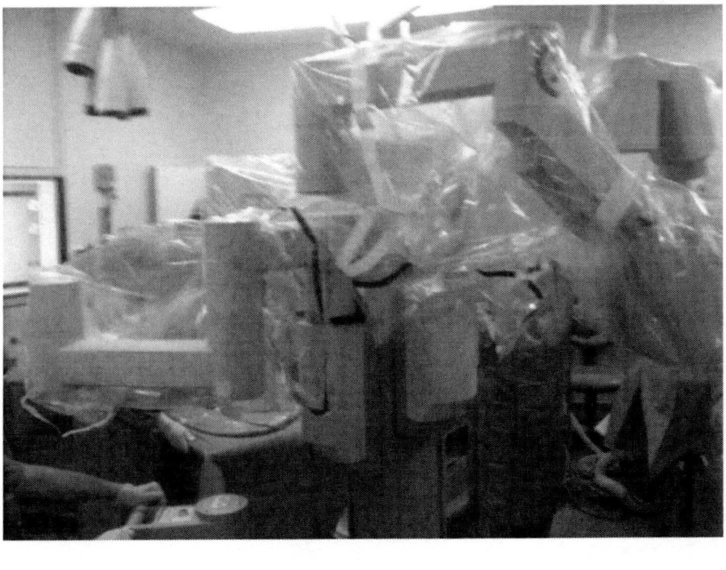

Driving the robot.

Care should be taken to avoid any injuries to the patient or desterilisation of the robotic arms. Special care should be taken on the robotic arm that is going to be attached on the left of the patient in order to be able to reach the trocar especially in obese patients. While docking, the team should also take into account the fact that the robotic arms should not have any obstacles to move especially in the area of the patient's legs while at the same time any injury in the patient should be avoided during the movements of the robotic arms.

The camera arm is the first one to be connected to the patient by locking the camera trocar mount to the camera trocar and using the camera setup joint buttons to move the camera arm into position and the camera clutch to adjust the final trajectory of the arm. The instrument arms are attached to the robotic trocars by using the port clutch for gross movements of the instrument arms and the instrument clutch for the final trajectory. As already noted, care must be taken to avoid collision, contact or pinching the patient's arm, body, or leg. The endoscope is inserted by placing the lens into the trocar and locking it into the camera trocar. Then it can be advanced into the surgical field using the camera clutch button. The EndoWristinstruments are inserted by straightening the instrument wrist and placing the instrument tip into the trocar and sliding the instrument housing into the adaptor and then advanced into the surgical field using the instrument clutch button under laparoscopic vision.

To remove an instrument, the surgeon should straighten the instrument wrist and then the assistant squeezes the release levers and pulls the instrument out. Please before removal have all the instruments under vision and take care of not holding any tissues.

Side Docking

For the gynaecological operations, usually the robot is docked at an approximately 45° angle to the lower torso, aligned with the outer border of the right stirrup. The rest of the patient and trocar setup is similar to traditional docking. The main benefit of side docking is better pelvic access.

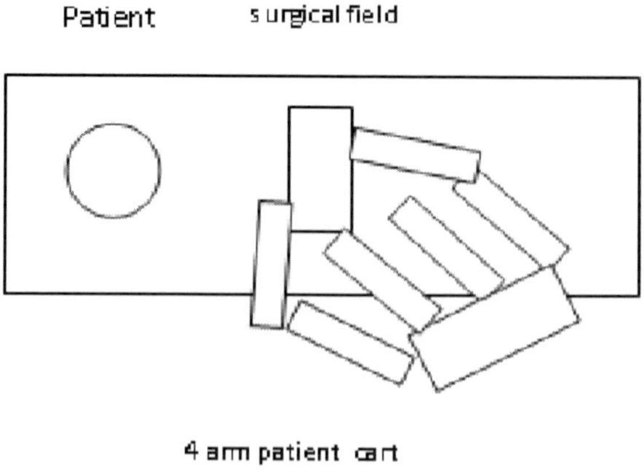

Side docking.

Once the robotic operation is completed, all instruments are removed first, followed by the endoscope. Then the arms are disconnected from the trocars. The patient cart is undocked and the sterile accessories and drapes are removed and the system is cleaned. It should be mentioned that it is not necessary to power the system off between surgical operations.

Correct patient and port placement is of pivotal importance because they permit adequate movement of robotic arms and assistance in order to avoid the chasing swords phenomenon. In cases of incorrect port placement, it is necessary to reposition one or more port(s) and redock the robotic arms, which could cause a subsequent increase in operative time.

Chapter 4

Role of the Nurse

The nurse team implicated in robotic procedures should be very well trained as they have the following significant roles:

a) identify the system's components and know how they are used
b) prepare the surgical system before surgery by connecting the proper cords from the video tower to the surgeon's console and from the robotic arms to the surgeon's console.

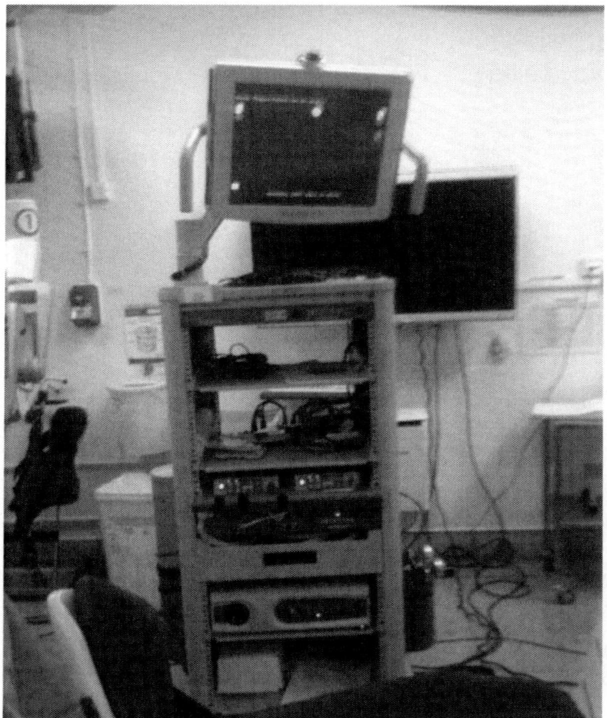

Video tower.

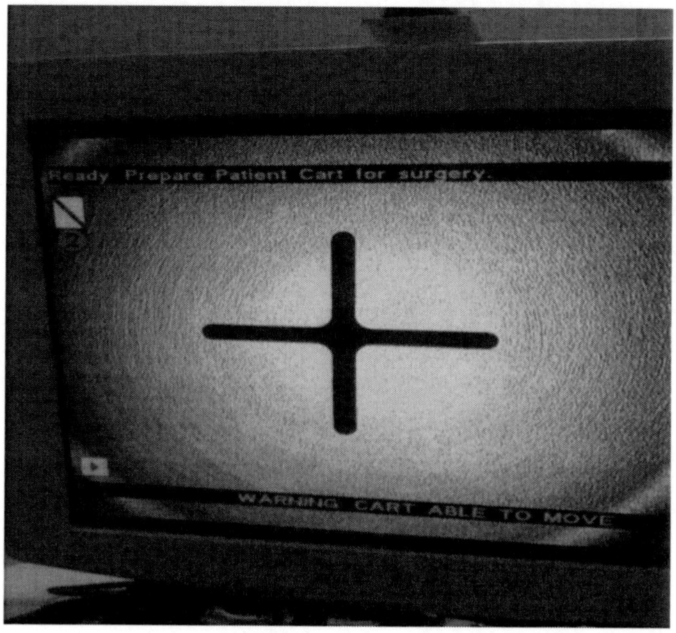
Ready Prepare Patient Cart for surgery.
WARNING CART ABLE TO MOVE

Aligning the camera.

a) Make sure that the surgical system's cords cannot be accidentally disconnected
b) inspect cords for any frayed areas or damage that could create an electrical hazard
c) ensure that the system is plugged into the proper electrical power outlets, then turn the system on and follow the instructions to home the system and place the surgical arms in a neutral position

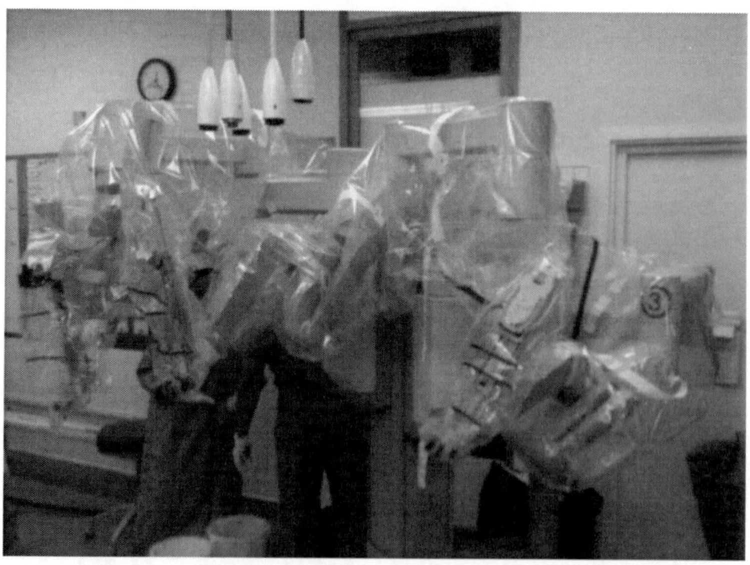

Sterile drapes on the robotic arms.

a) cover the robotic arms with sterile drapes

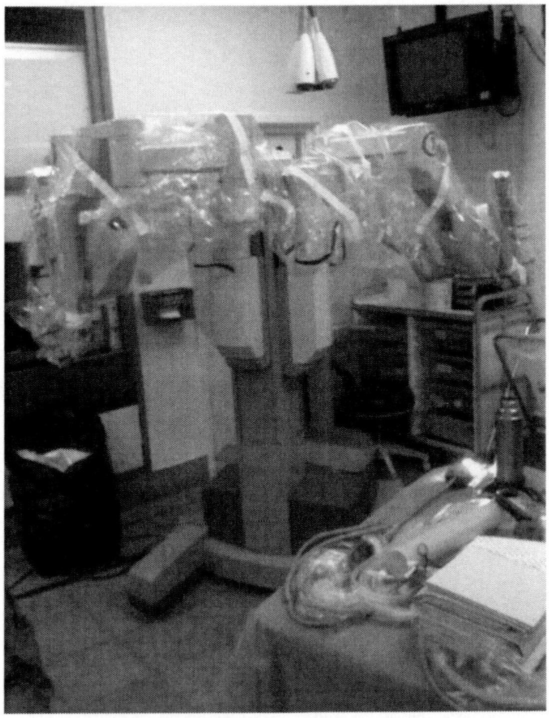

Preparation of the system.

b) prepare the unsterile camera and sterile scope

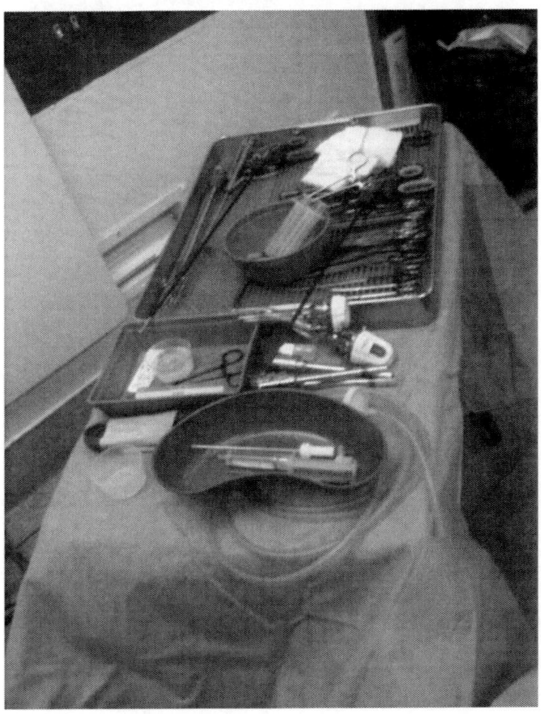

Preparation of the instruments.

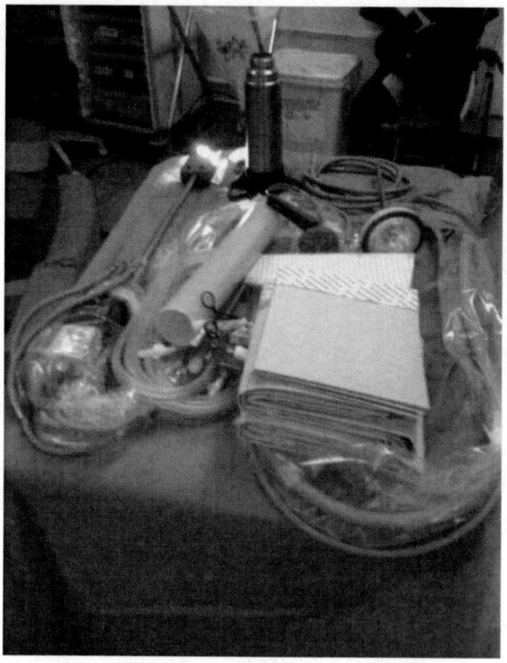

Preparation of the instruments.

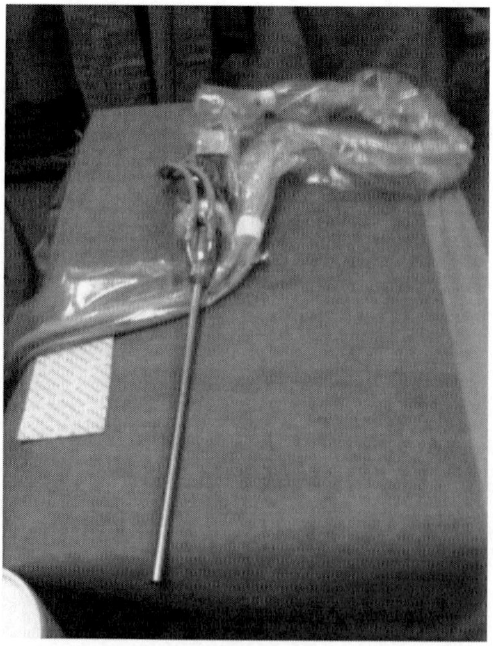

Preparation of the camera.

a) inspect the instruments for damage and replace damaged instruments
b) know the location of the emergency hex wrench that comes with the equipment because in case of a system failure, this wrench would free the surgical arms from the trocars

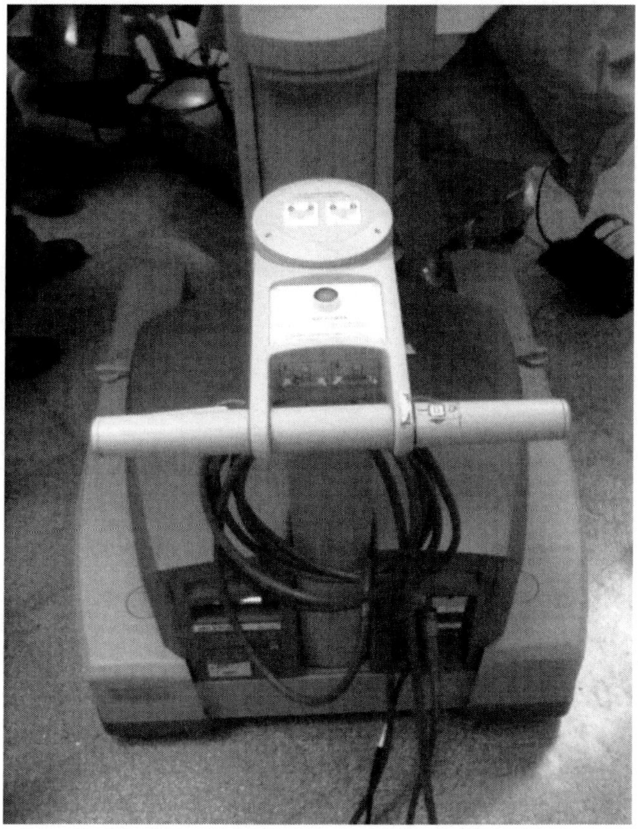

Drive the system.

a) place the system in position for patient docking
b) report any faults or system errors
c) before surgery, make sure the patient has given informed consent
d) when docking ensure that the robotic arms or cords are not resting on any part of the patient's body (safe patient positioning)
e) prevent nerve damage or loss of circulation in the arms by appropriately padding them
f) keep track of the number of times each robotic instrument is used
g) sterilize new instruments as needed

Chapter 5

The Role of Surgical Assistant in Robotic Procedures

The surgical assistant in robotic procedures has multiple roles and should be well trained. He/she is involved in the following:

a. Patient set up to semi-lithotomy position on Allen stirrups with the arm loosely tucked bilaterally

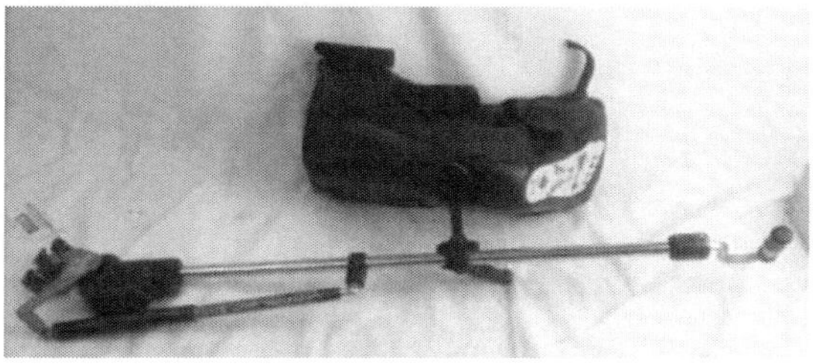

Allen stirrup.

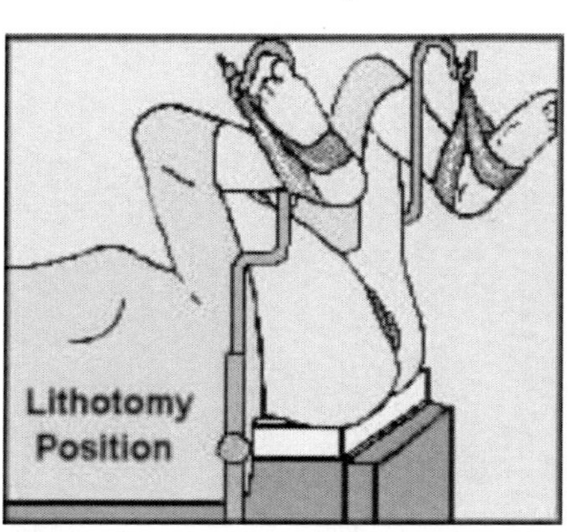

Lithotomy position.

b. Securing that the patient is on antiskid foam material

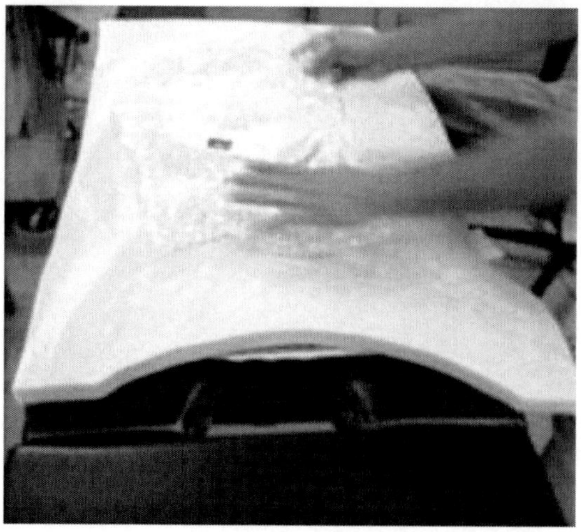

Matress.

c. Antisepsis

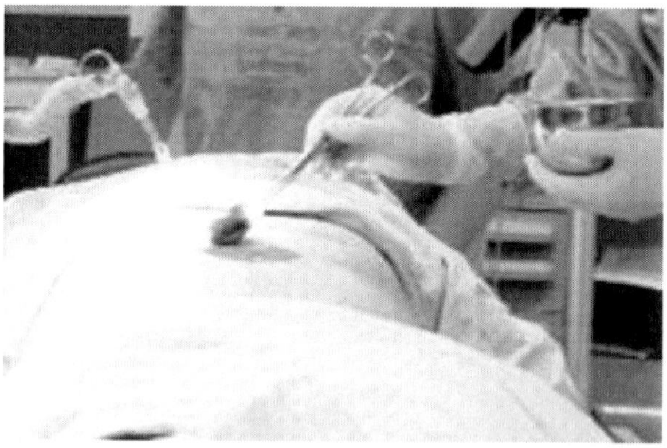

Preparing the abdomen.

d. Uterine manipulator insertion

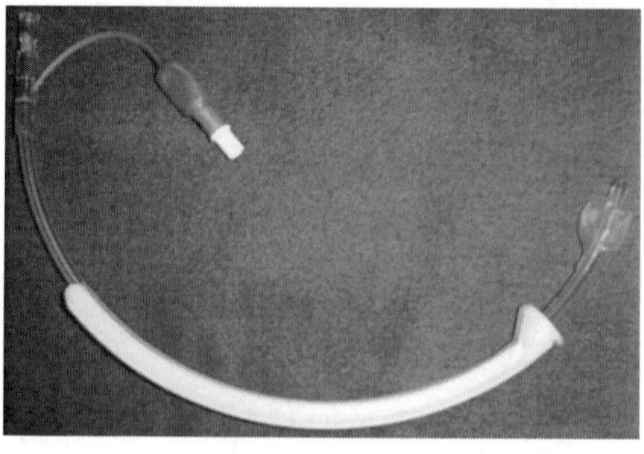

ZUMI® uterine manipulator.

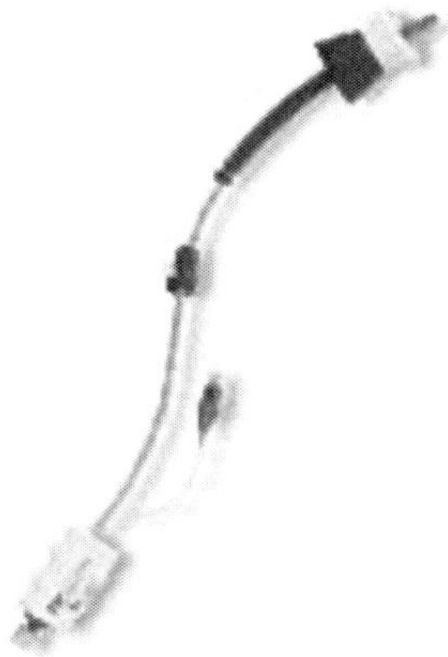

V-care uterine manipulator.

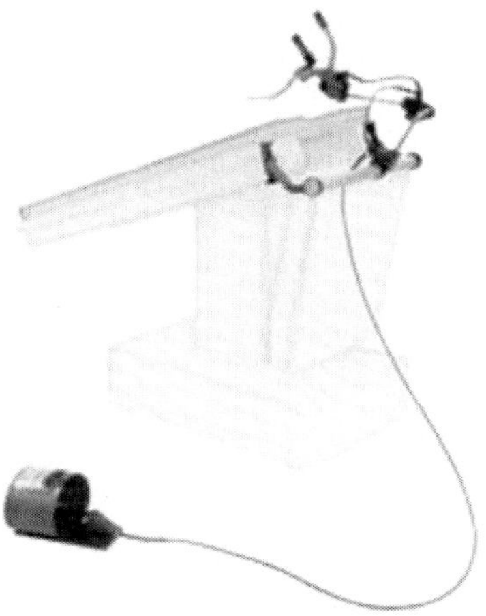

Uterine Positioning System™ (UPS) and the RUMI® or RUMI Arch™ uterine manipulators.

e. Docking and instrumentation

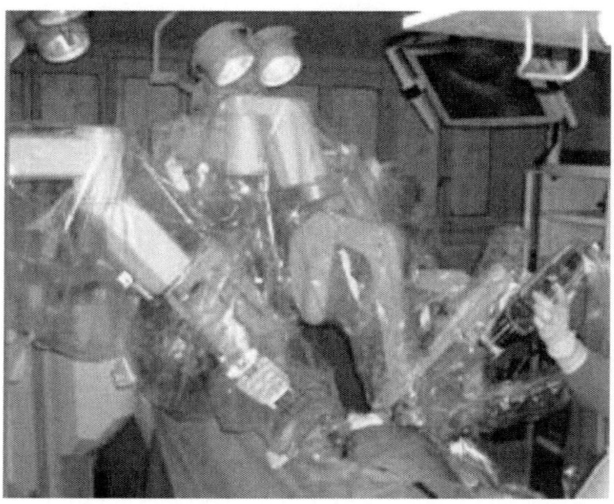

Docking.

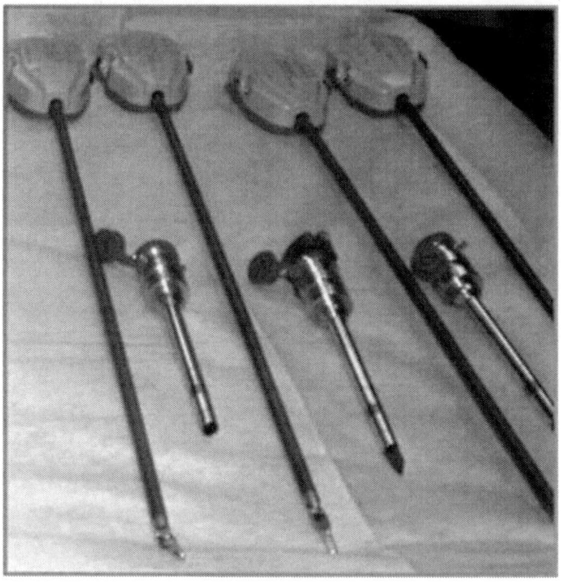

Instrumentation.

f. Sits to the left of the patient
g. Peritoneal cytology - Suction and irrigation
h. Removal of small specimens through the port
i. Tissue retraction
j. Insertion and removal of sutures

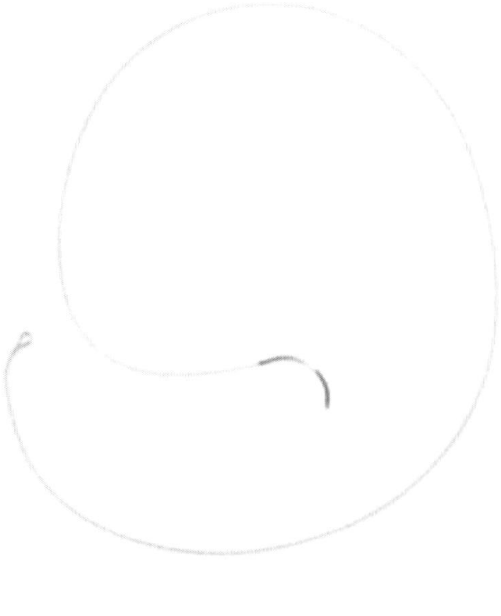

V-Loc suture.

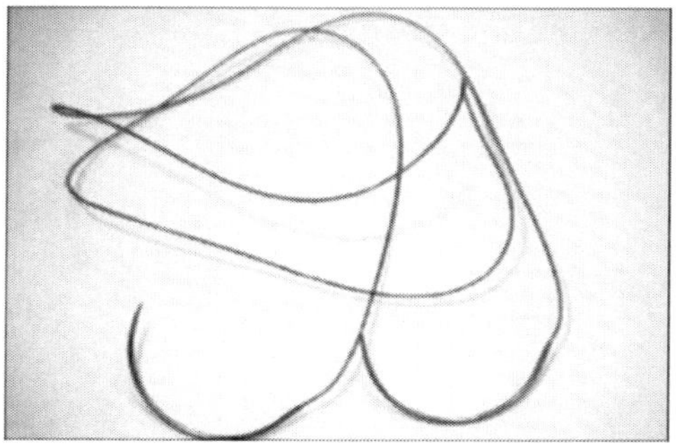

Quill Barbed Suture.

k. Cleaning the lens of the laparoscope

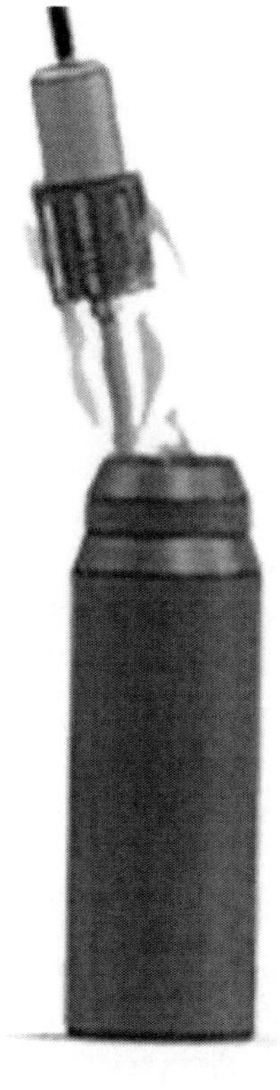

Scope Cleaning.

l. If there is no second assistant, by changing gloves:

- Uterine manipulation
- Maintains pneumoperitoneum after vaginal resection (usually by using a swab in a glove)
- Removal of the specimens vaginally

m. Undocking

Chapter 6

Robot Assisted Hysterectomy Set

Instruments

General set

Laparoscopic set including Scissors and Johann's

Gynae set/Hysteroscope set/D&C set

Da Vinci basic set

Da Vinci instrument set

Da Vinci light lead

Da Vinci scope warmer

Da Vinci Fenestrated bipolar forcep

Da Vinci Maryland/Cadiere forcep

Da Vinci monopolar sciscors

Sims retractor

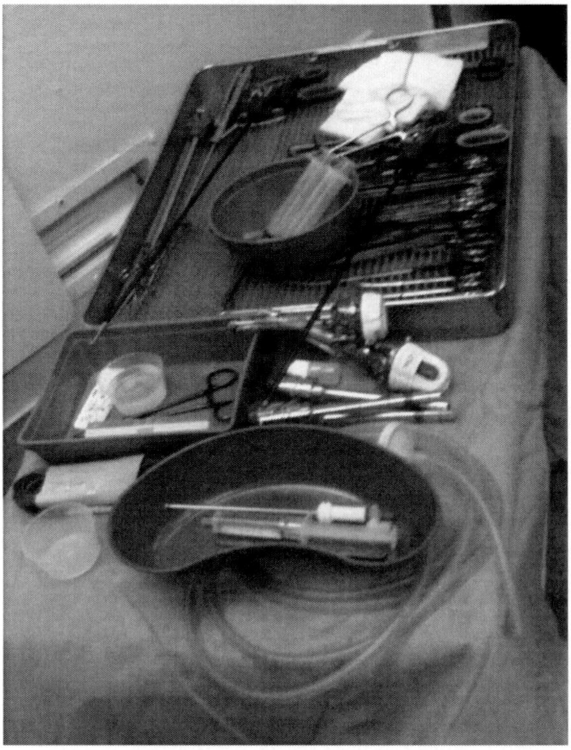

Laparoscopic set.

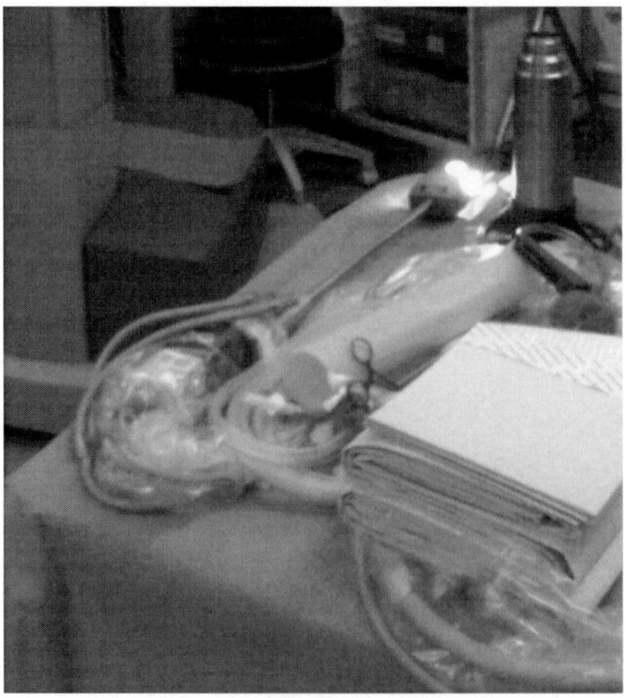

Robotic camera.

Gynaecological Robotic Complete Box

Da Vinci port/cannula seal 10/12 mm x 3

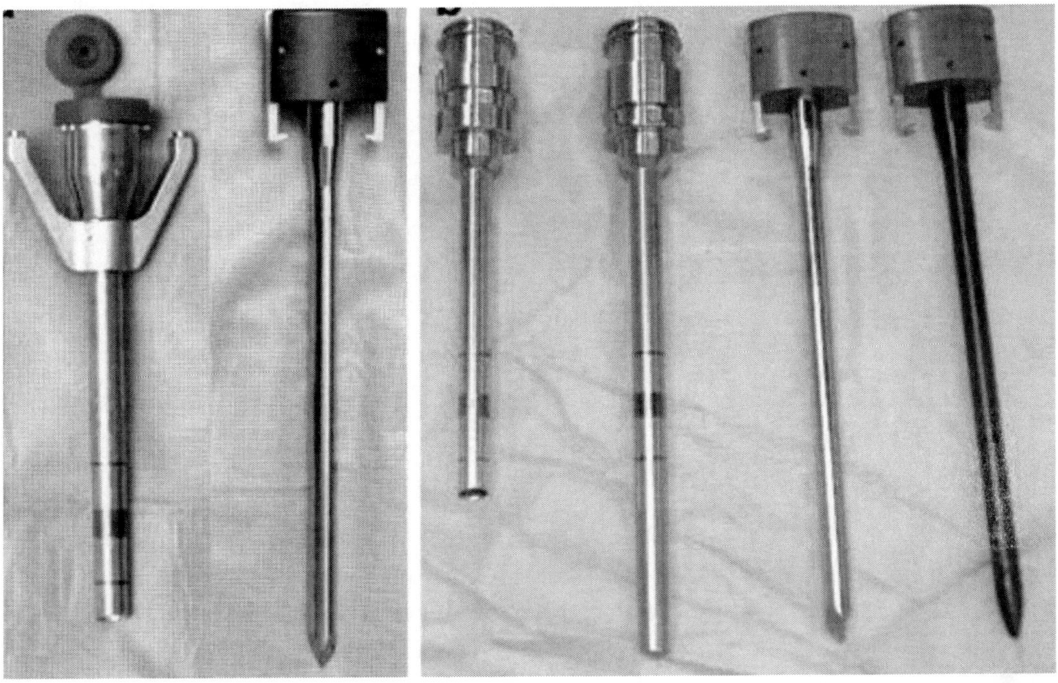

Da Vinci trocars.

Intuitive tip cover accessory x 1

Applied medical scope warmer seal x 1

Electrolube antistick solution x 1

Insufflation tubing x 1

Da Vinci robot arm drapes:

- instrument arm drape x 3
- camera arm drape x 1
- camera head drape x 1

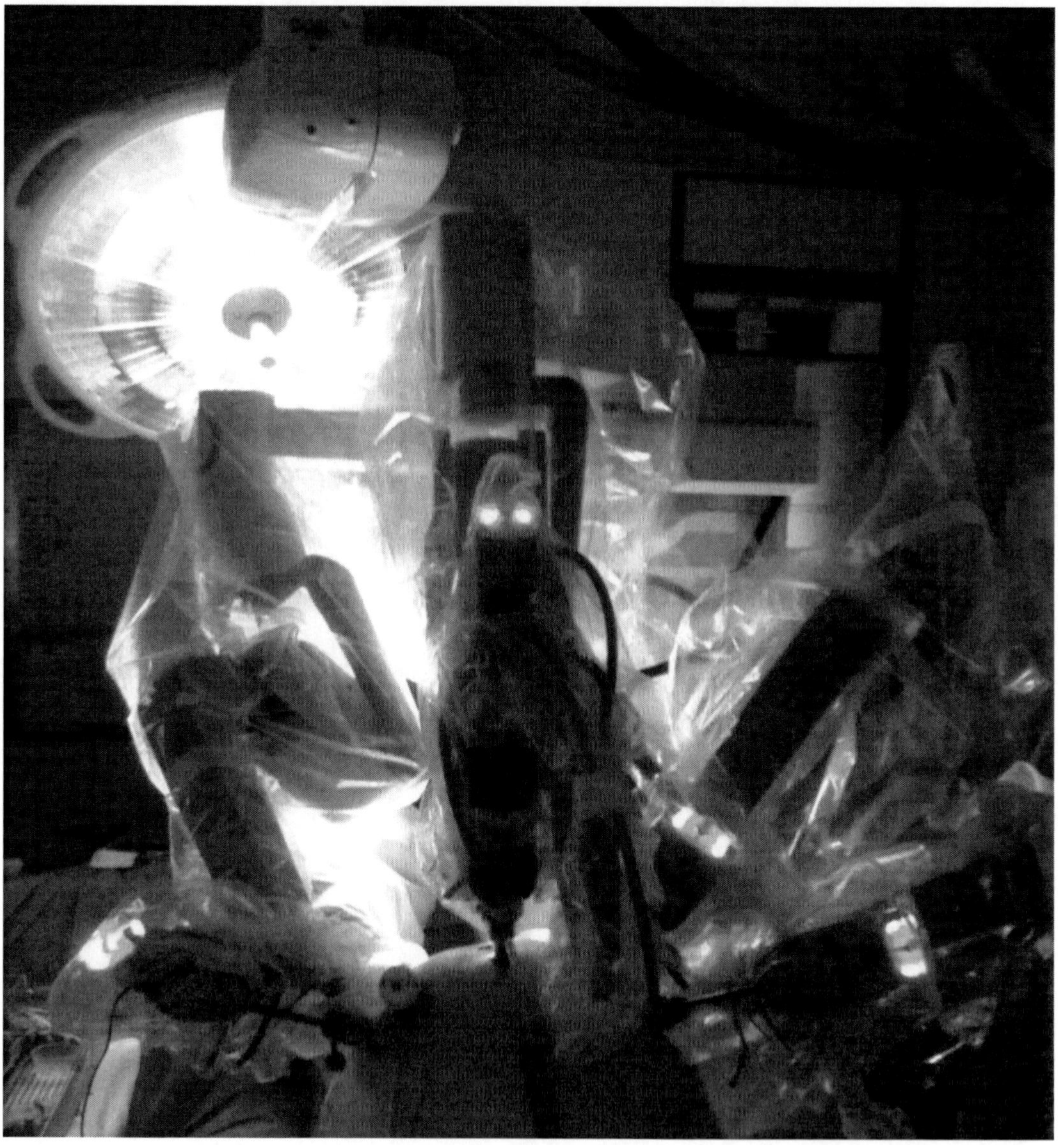

Docked robot.

Ethicon bladeless trocar x 1
Insufflation needle x 1
Core trumpet x 1
Smoke venting filter x 1

EndoWrist® Instruments commonly used for gynaecological operations:

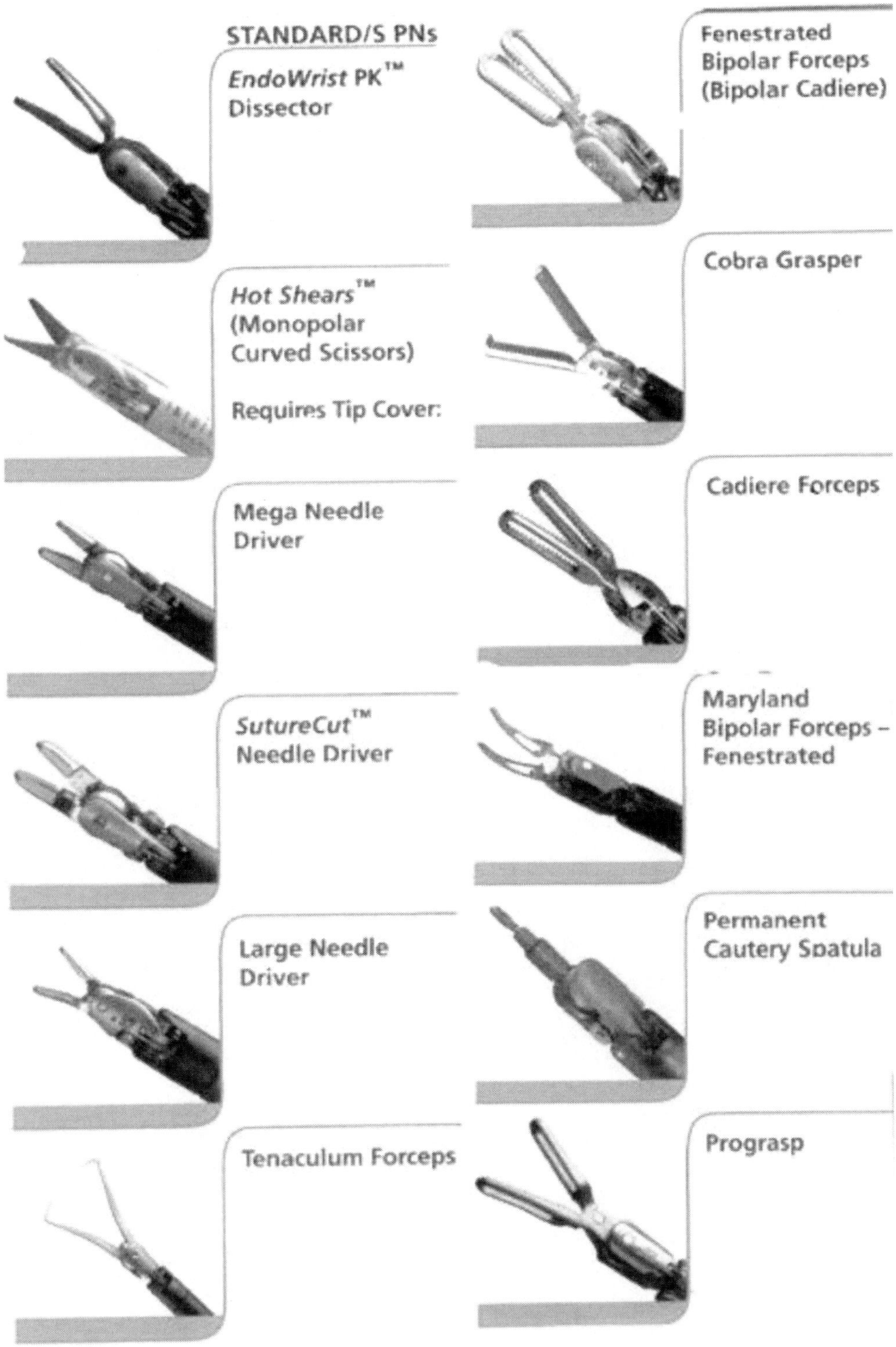

Intuitive instruments.

Skin Preparation

Betadine or other solution

Catheter set

Catheter pack
Size 16 catheter
Urometer
Travasept
Instillagel

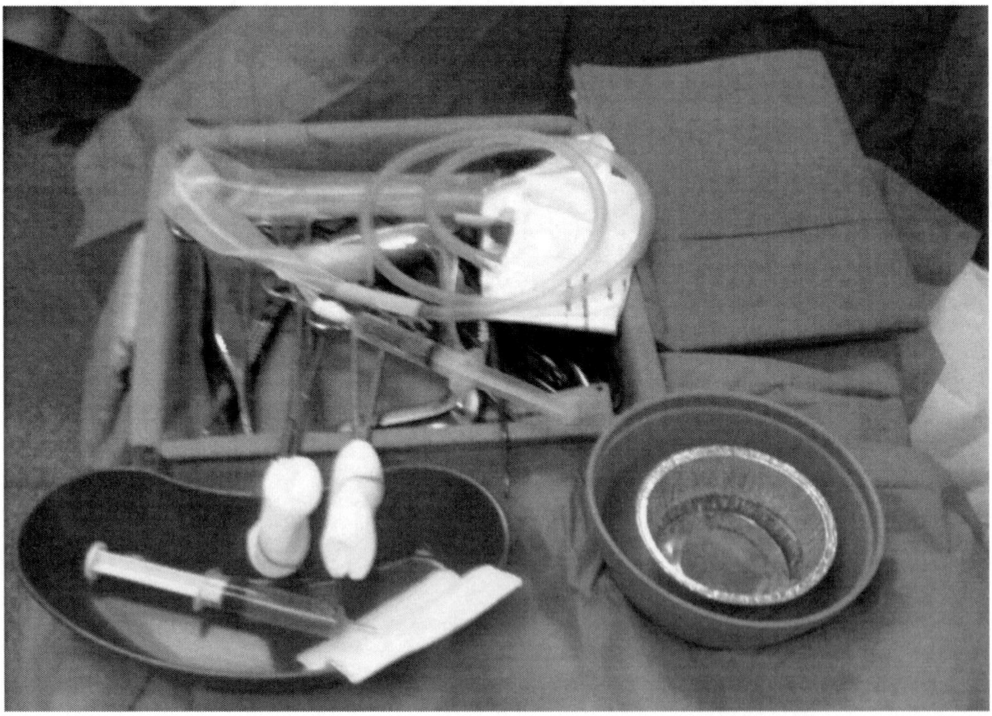

Catheter set.

Drapes

Universal drape
Lithotomy drape

Swabs

4x3=10
9x9=5
Tonsil swabs x 5

Local infiltration

20 mls of Marcain 0.25% with adrenaline 1:200,000 x 2

Blades

Size 11 blade x 1

Sutures

Vicryl 1 x 1
Monocryl 3-0 on a cutting needle x 1
PDS 1 J shape x 1
Monocryl 0 X 1
V-loc 2-0 suture or other barbed suture x 1

Clips

Haemaloc clips

Uterine manipulator

V-care or other uterine manipulator

Disposables

Hug-u-vac and long gel pad
Receivers, gallipots and bowl liner
Lap diathermy bag
Light handles
20 ml syringe x 2
Green hypo
Red hypo
Retrieval bag x 1
Floseal
Surgicel

Dressings

Opsites baby x 4
Skin glue

Chapter 7

Instruments

(Names and photos):

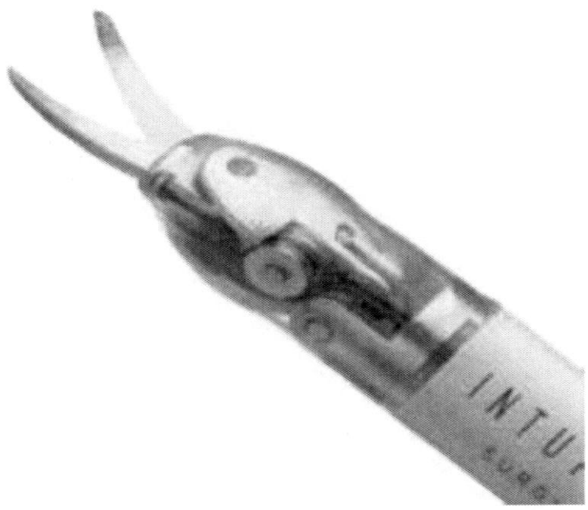

Hot Shears™

(Monopolar Curved Scissors).

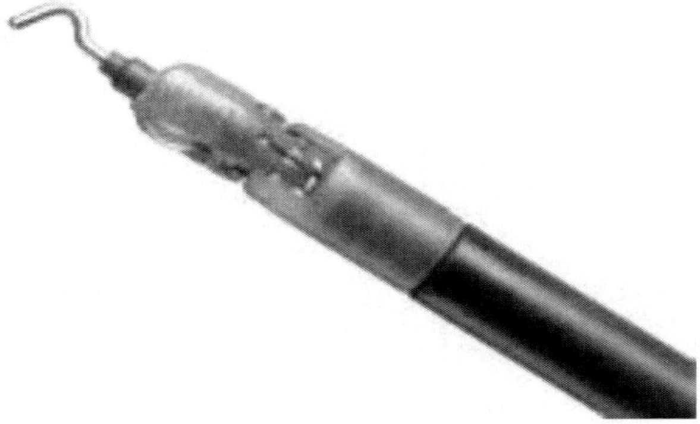

Permanent

Cautery Hook.

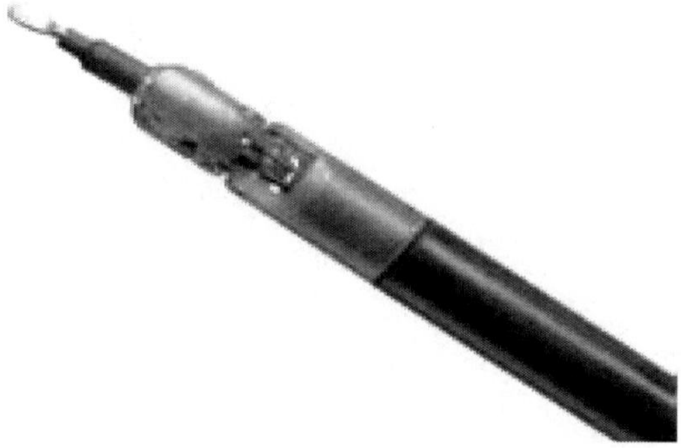

Permanent

Cautery Spatula.

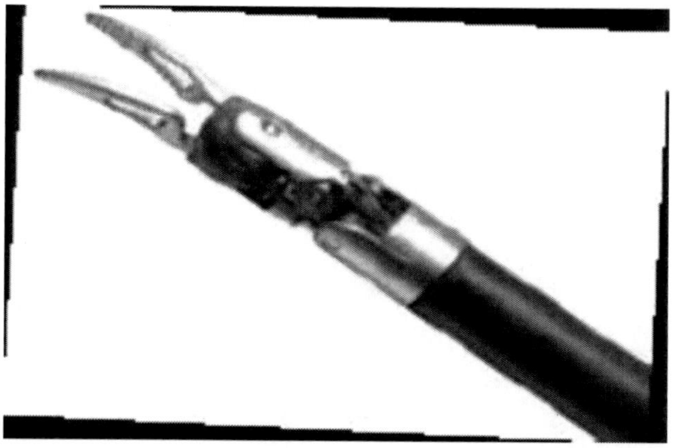

Maryland Bipolar Forceps.

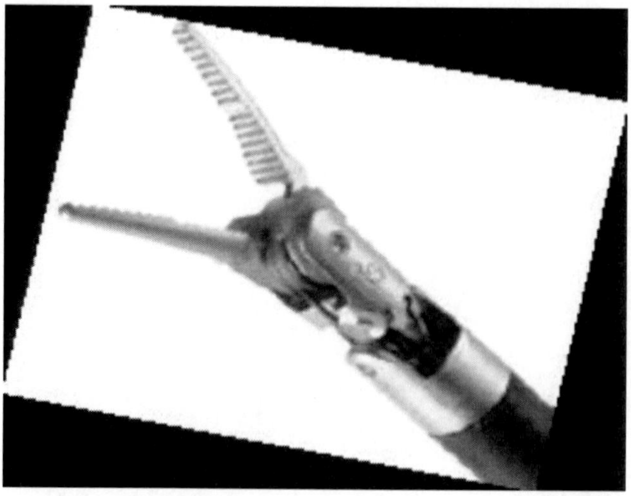

PK® Dissecting Forceps.

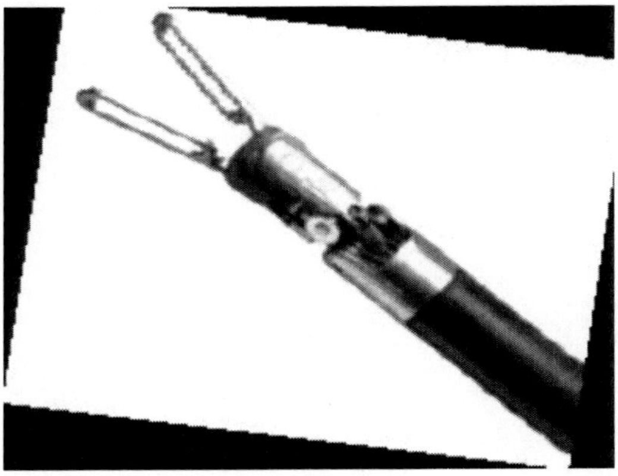

Fenestrated

Bipolar Forceps.

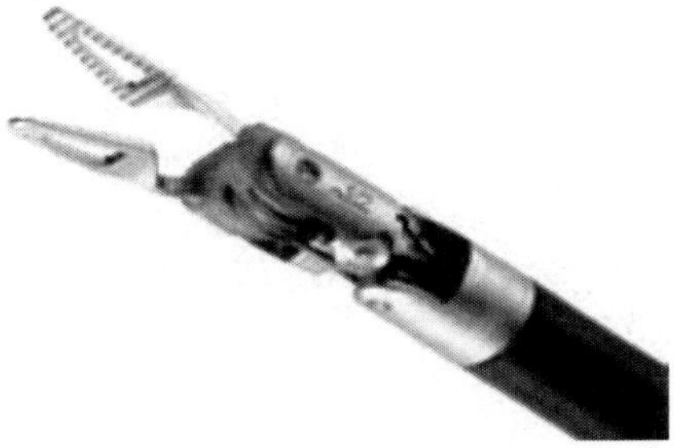

PreCise™ Bipolar Forceps.

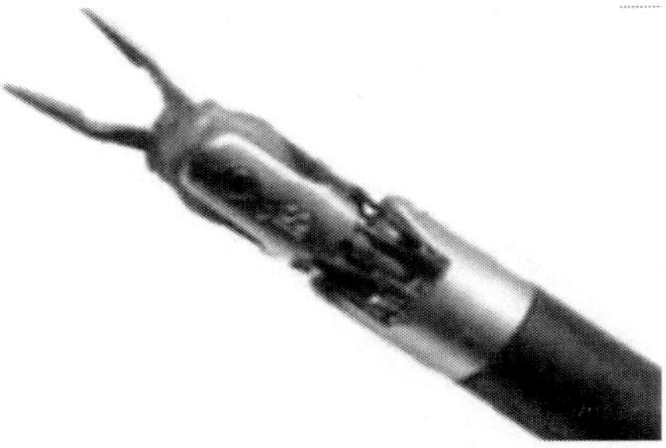

Micro Bipolar Forceps.

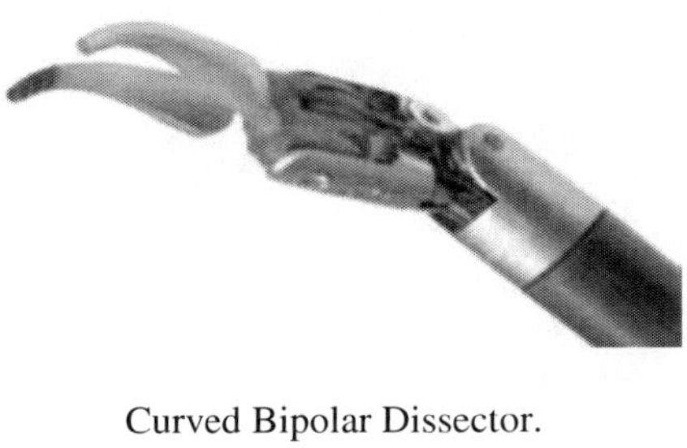

Curved Bipolar Dissector.

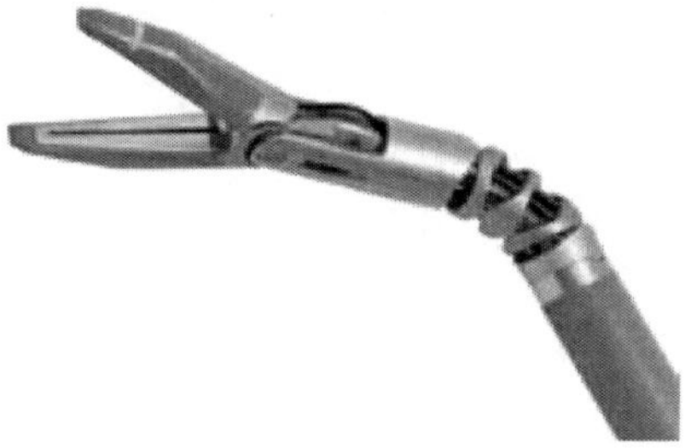

Vessel Sealer.

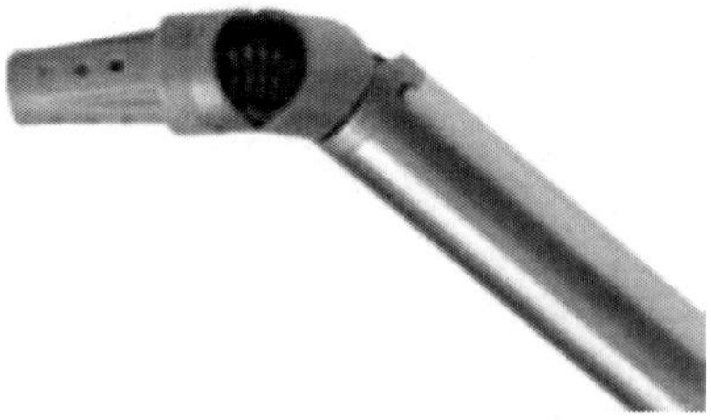

Suction / Irrigator.

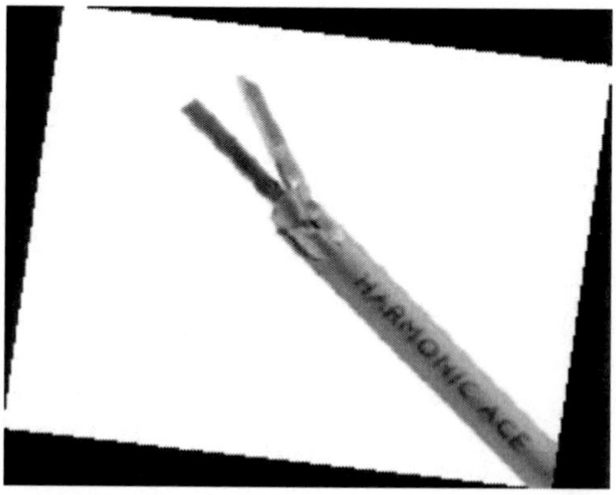

Harmonic ACE® Curved Shears.

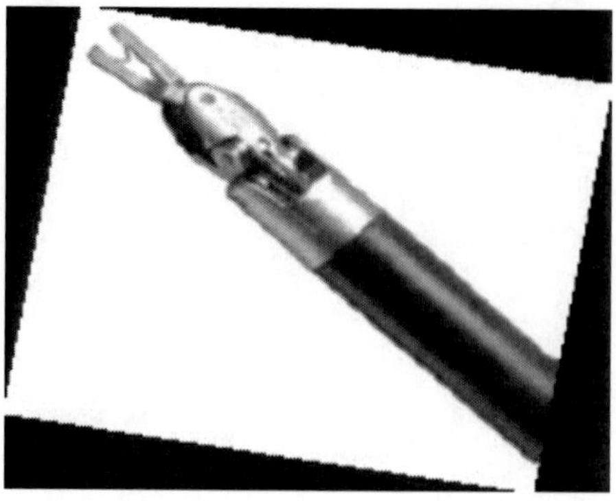

Small

Clip Applier.

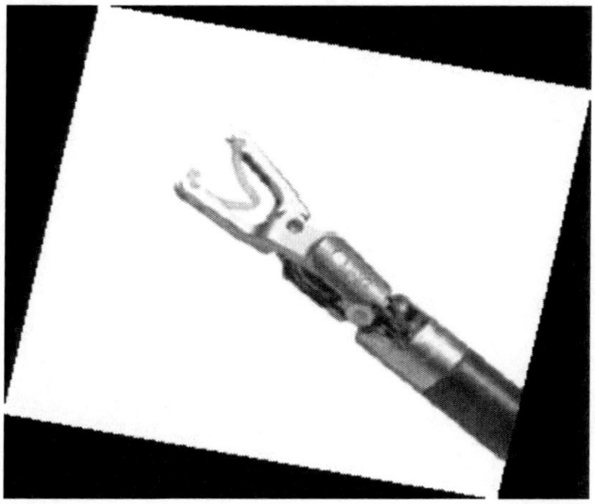

Medium-Large

Clip Applier.

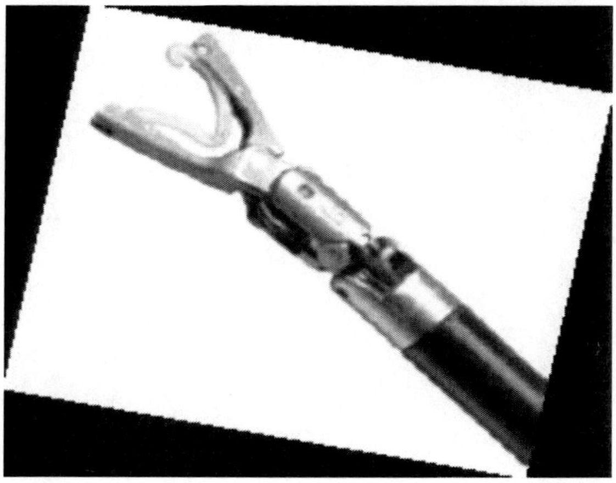

Large

Clip Applier.

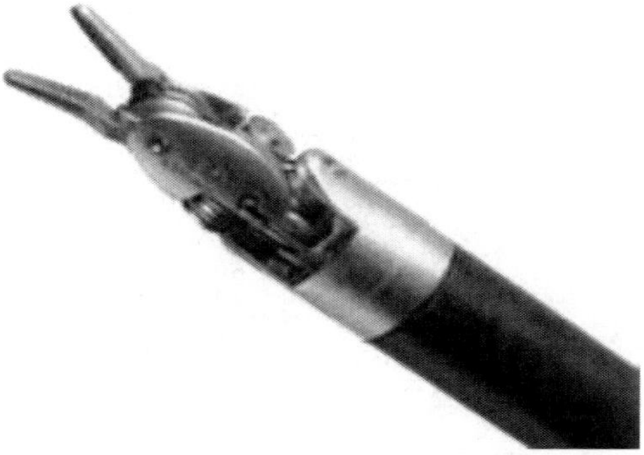

Large Needle Driver.

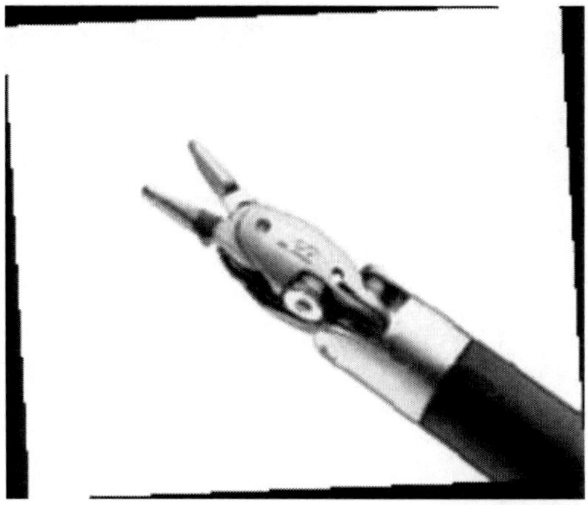

Large Suture Cut ™

Needle D river.

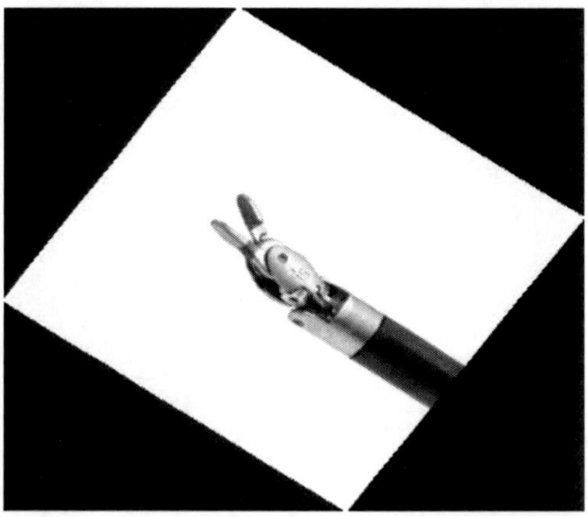

Mega Suture Cut™

Needle Driver.

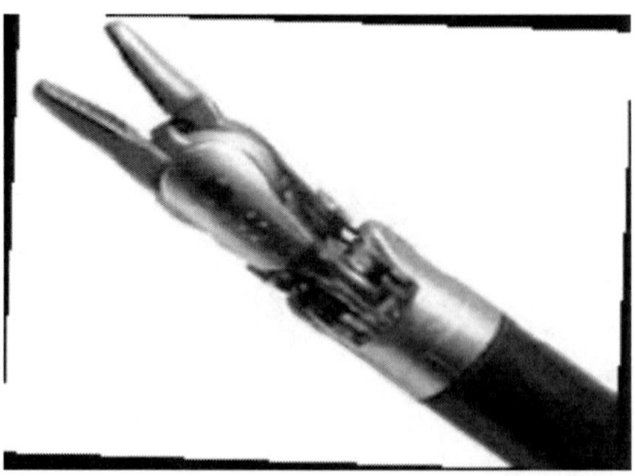

Mega™ Needle Driver.

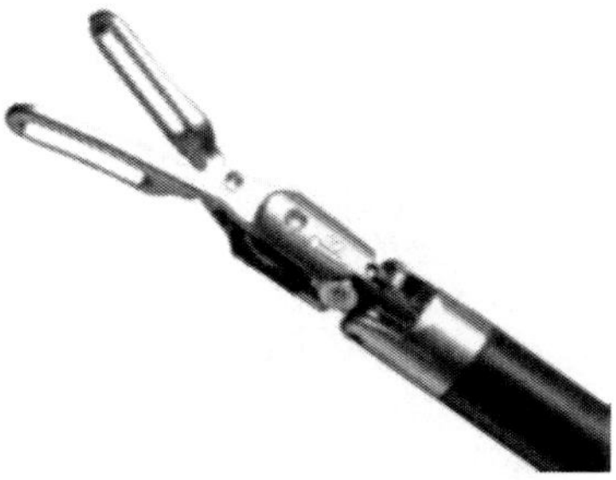

ProGrasp™ Forceps.

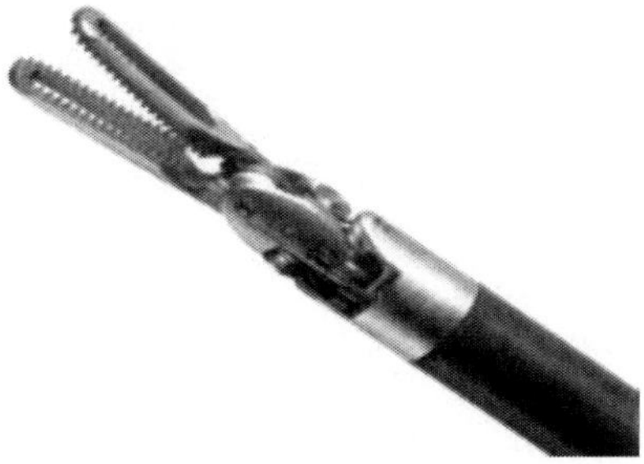

Cadiere Forceps.

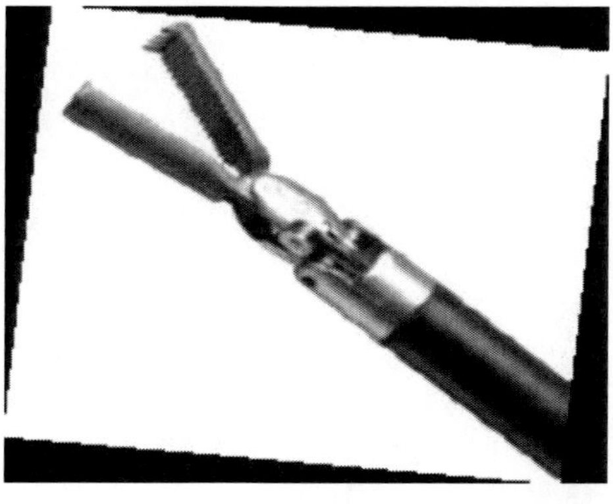

Cobra Grasper.

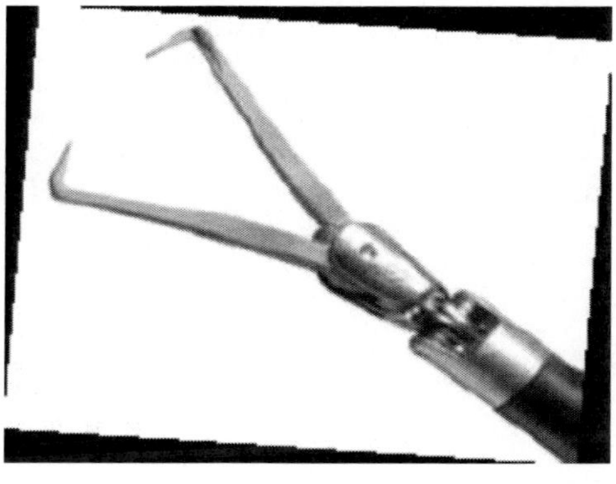

Tenaculum Forceps.

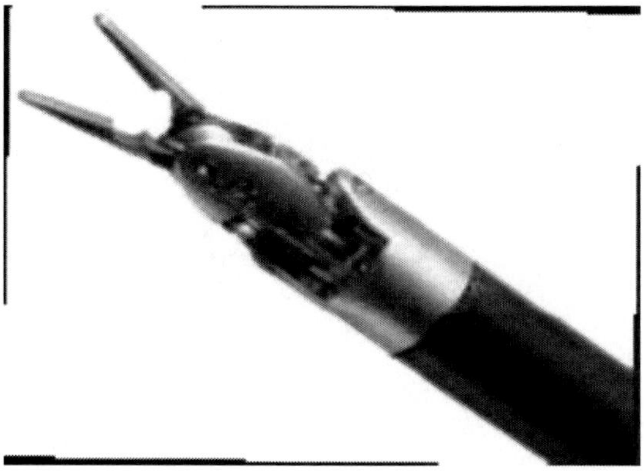

DeBakey Forceps.

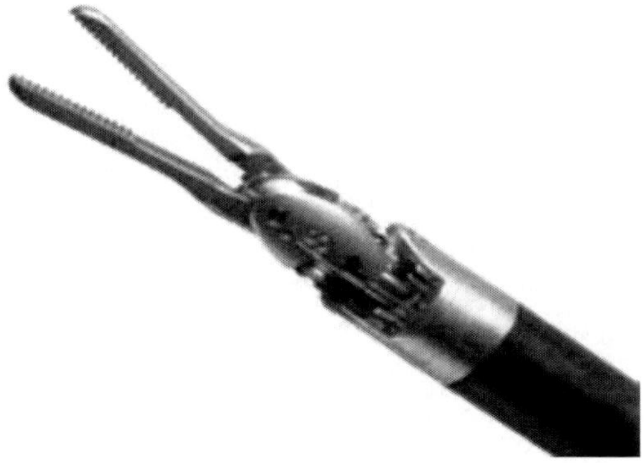

Long Tip Forceps.

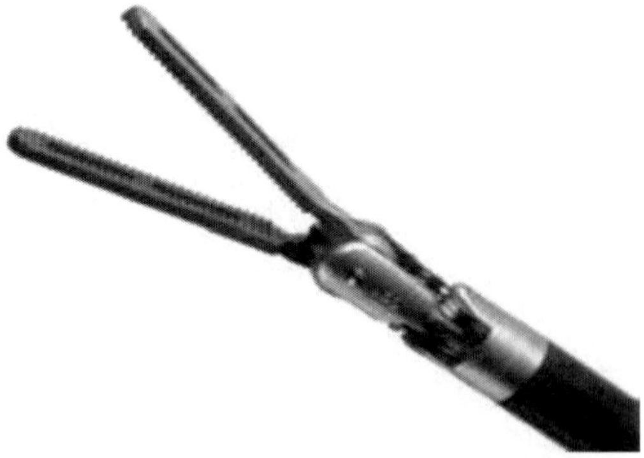

Double Fenestrated

Grasper.

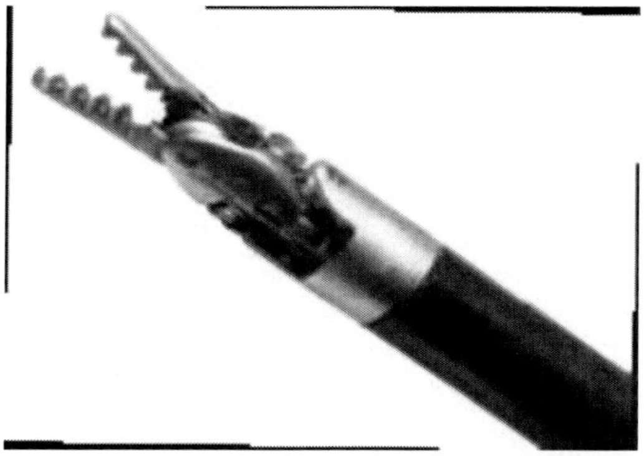

Resano Forceps.

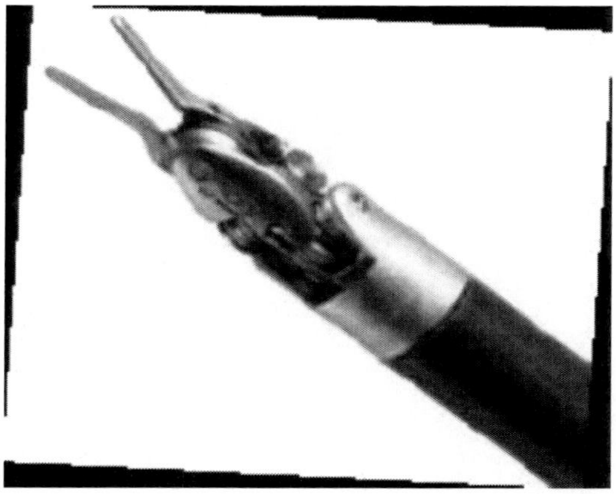

Fine Tissue Forceps.

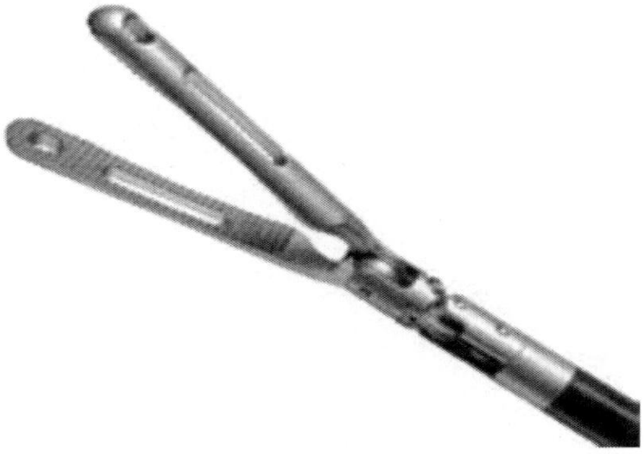

Graptor™

(Grasping Retractor).

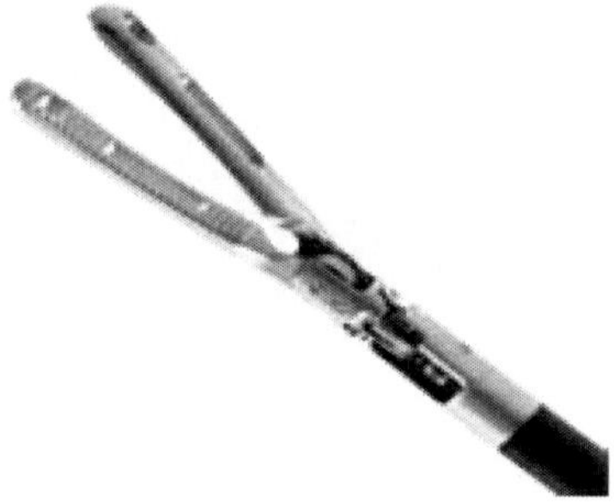

Small Graptor™

(Grasping Retractor).

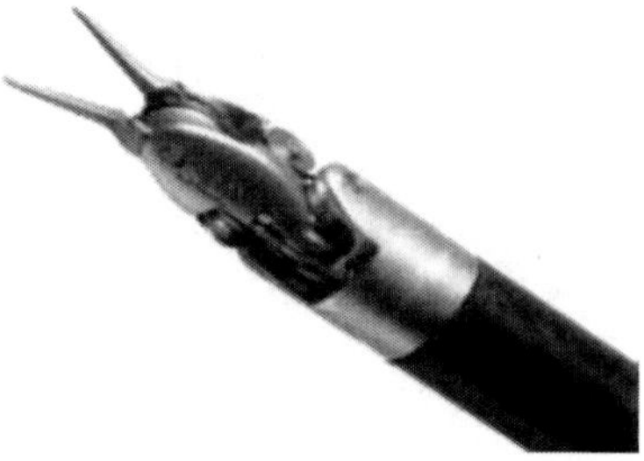

Black Diamond

Micro Forceps.

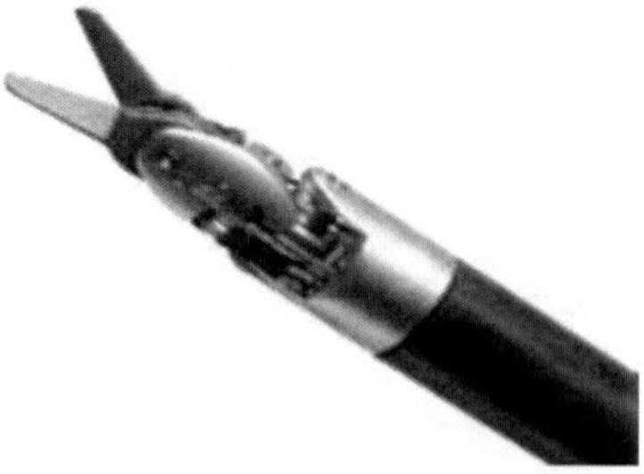

Round Tip Scissors.

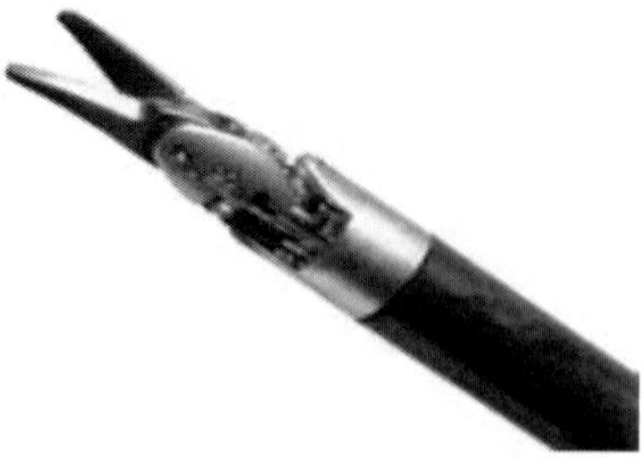

Curved Scissors.

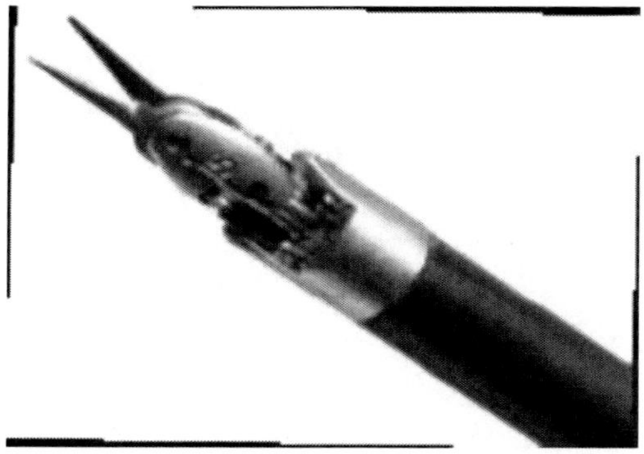

Potts Scissors.

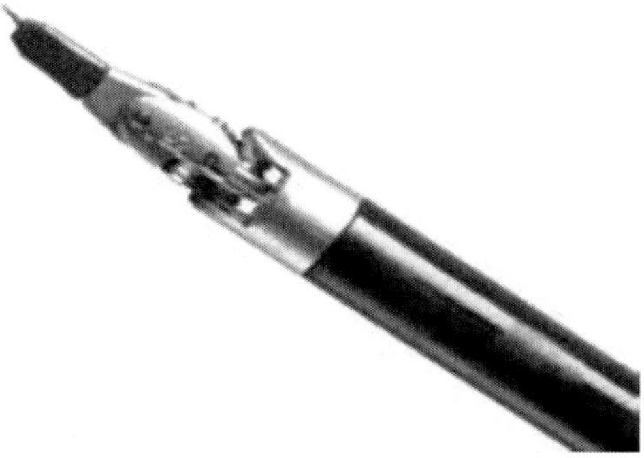

Snap-_t™

Scalpel

Instrument.

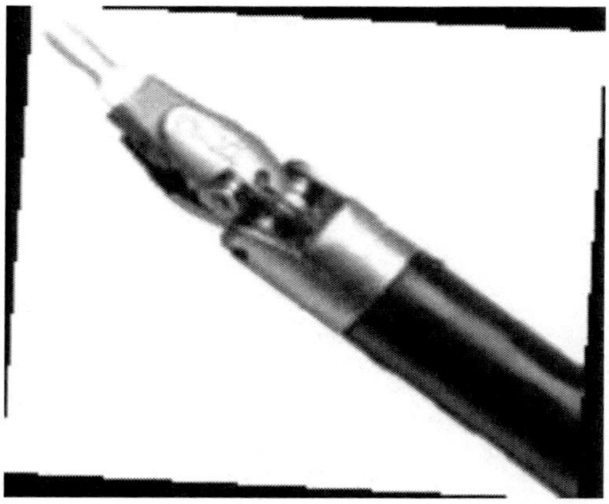

Snap-_t™

Scalpel

Instrument.

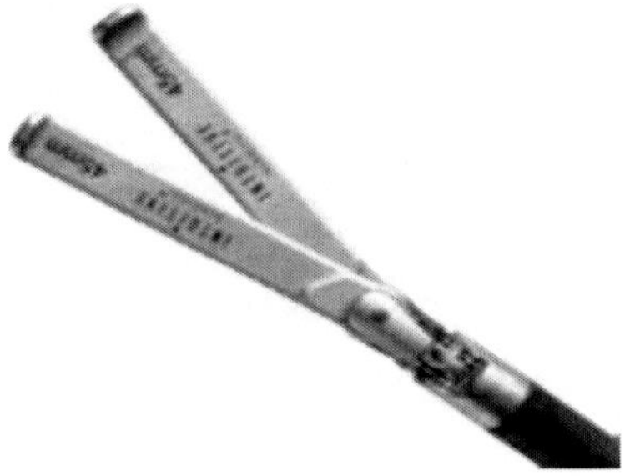

Atrial Retractor.

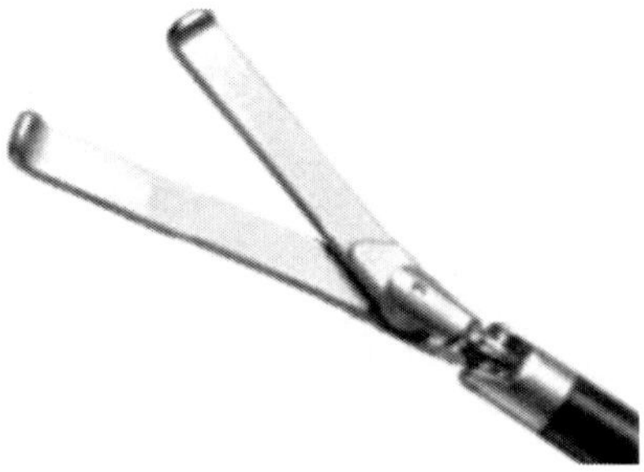

Atrial Retractor

Short Right.

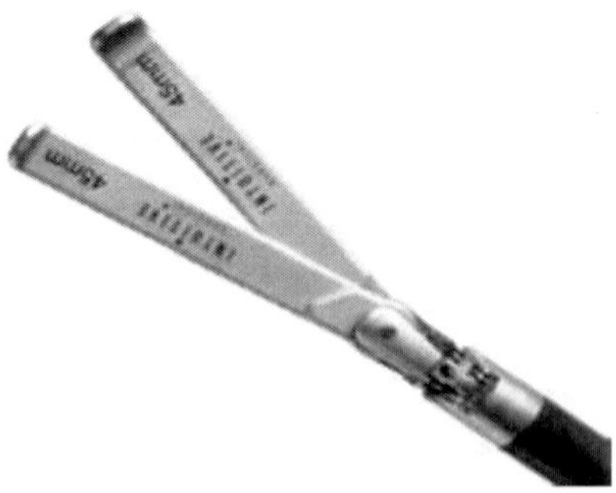

Dual Blade Retractor.

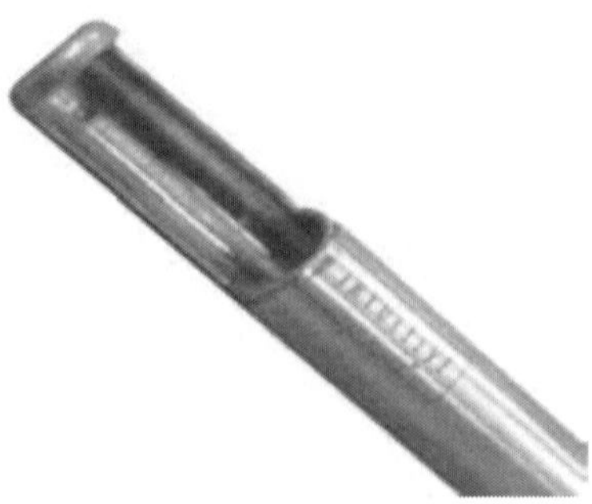

EndoPass

Delivery Instrument.

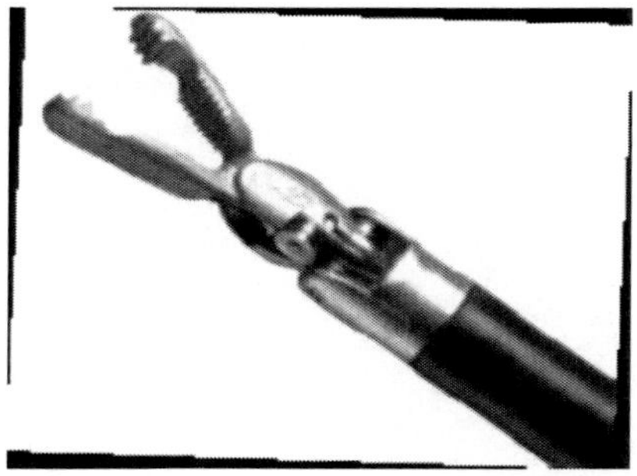

Cardiac Probe Grasper.

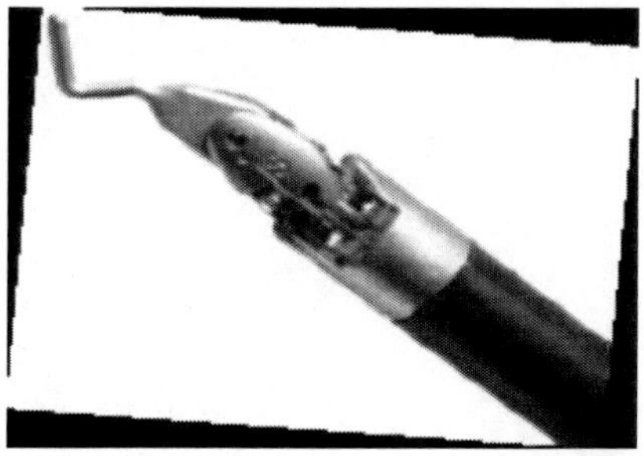

Valve Hook.

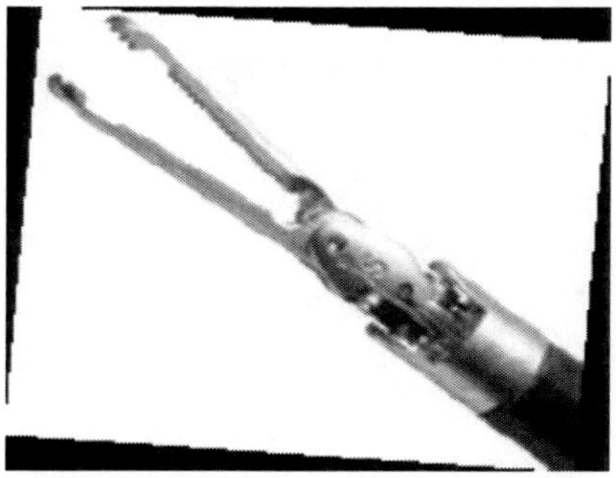

Pericardial Dissector.

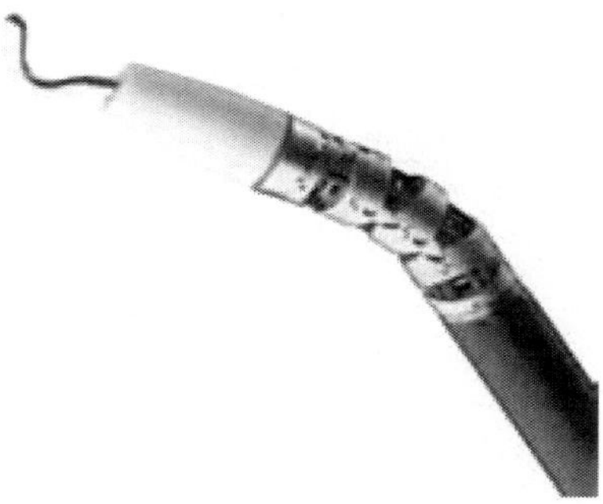

Monopolar Cautery.

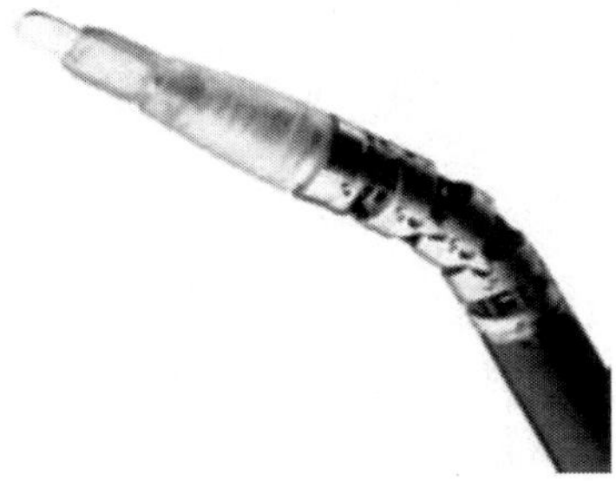

Monopolar Cautery.

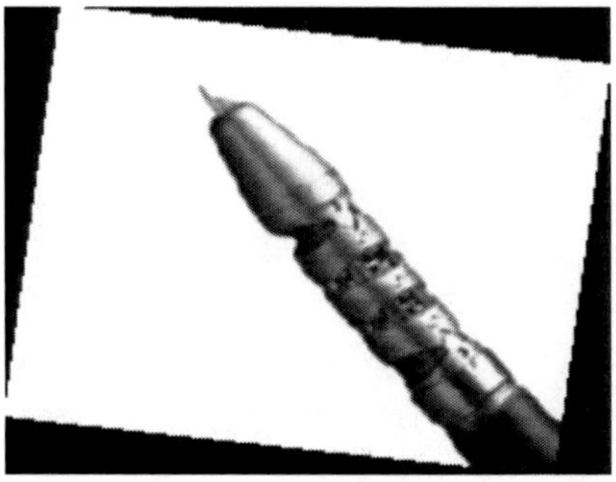

5 Fr. Introducer.

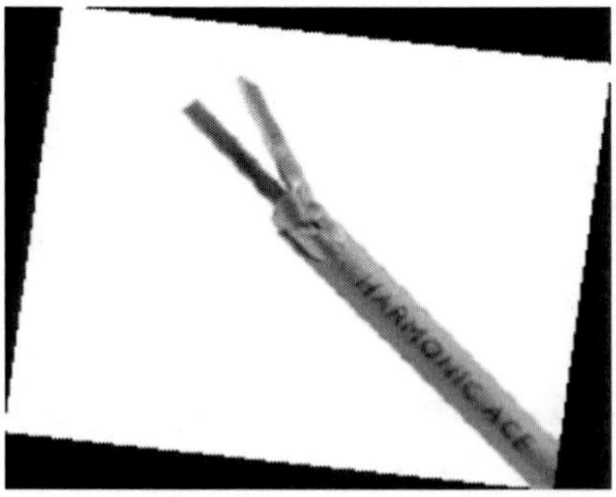

Harmonic ACE® Curved Shears.

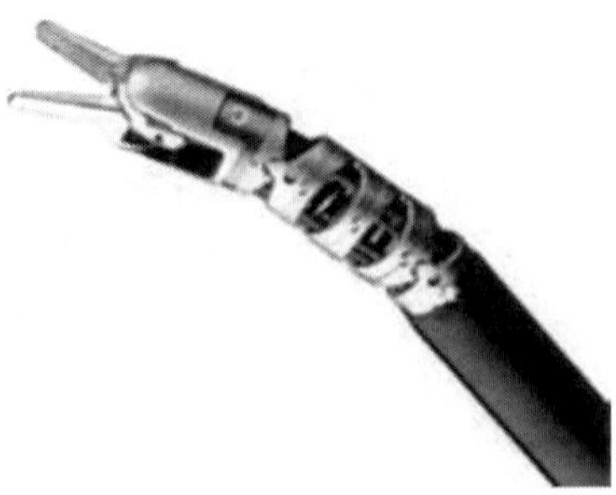

Needle Driver.

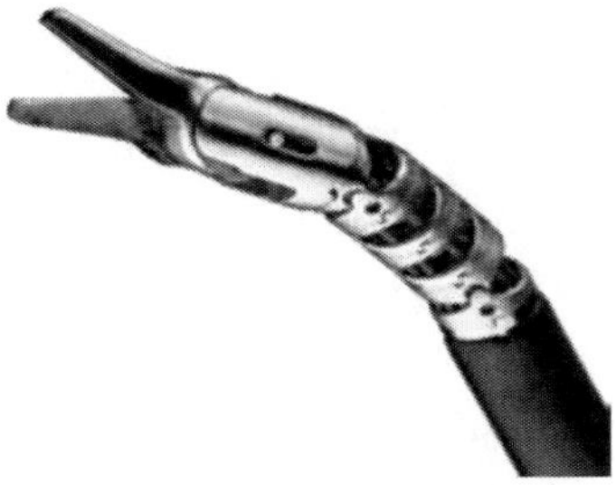

Round Tip Scissors.

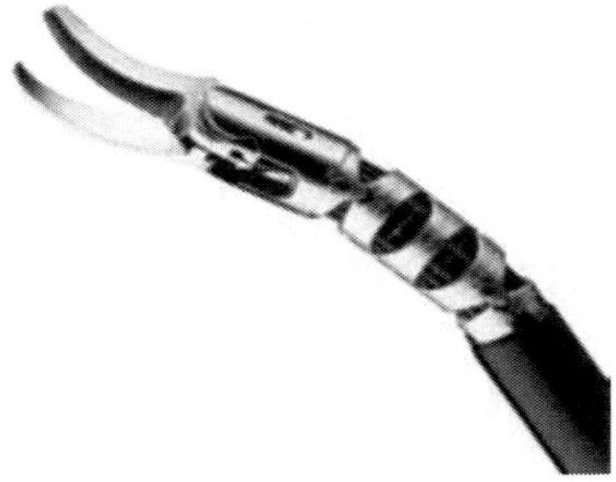

Curved Scissors.

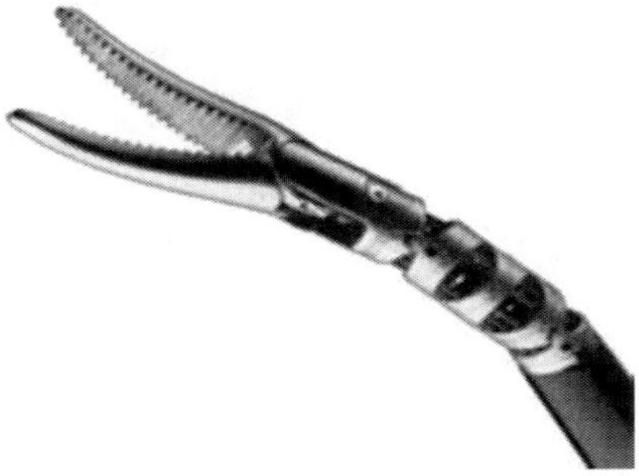

Maryland Dissector.

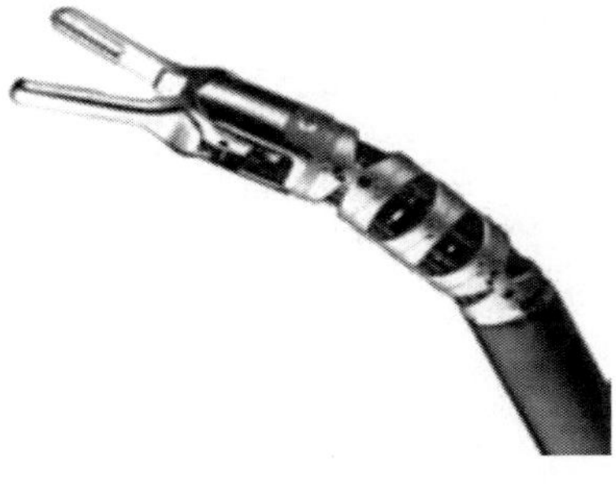

DeBakey Forceps.

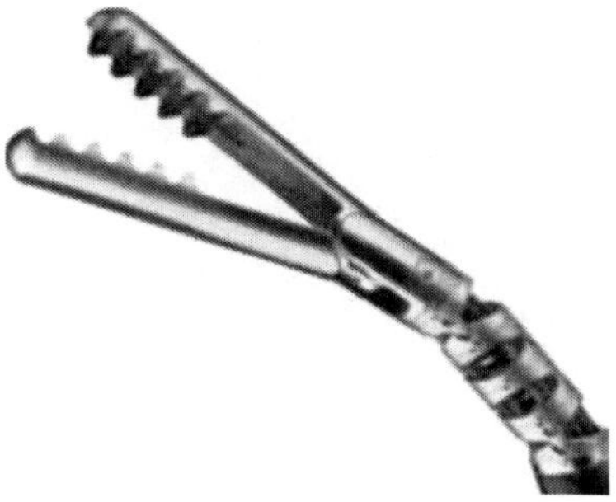

Schertel Grasper.

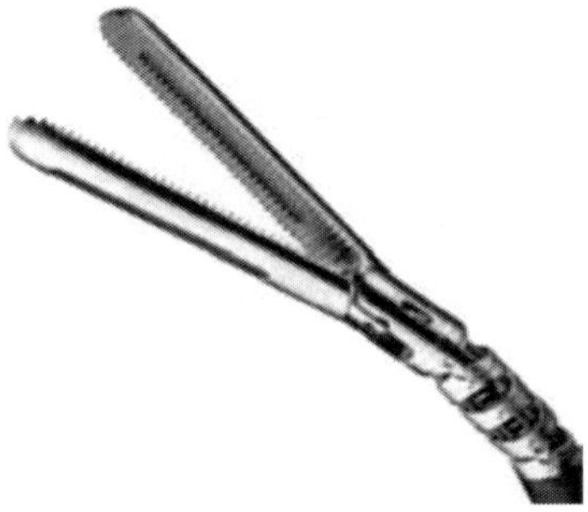

Bowel Grasper.

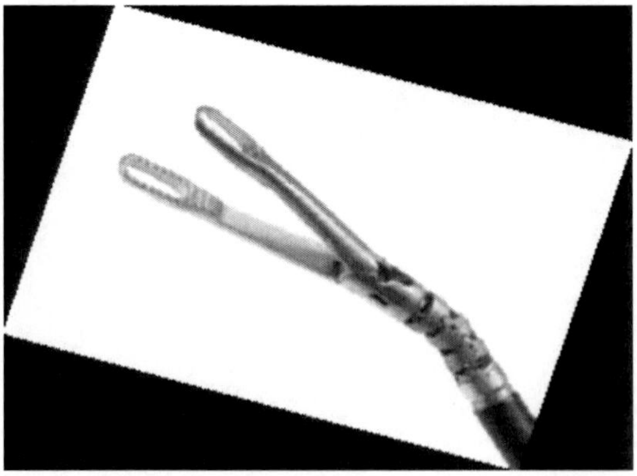

Thoracic Grasper.

Chapter 8

Veress and Trocars Insertion

Pre-Insertion Risk Evaluation

The safety of inserting a Veress needle or port into the peritoneal cavity depends on mobility of the underlying viscera. So it is wise to exclude the possibility of intraabdominal adhesions between underlying bowel and anterior abdominal wall by careful review of past medical, surgical history in the notes including history of post-operative peritonitis, endometriosis or PID.

Careful abdominal examination preoperatively can reveal abdominal surgical scars and clarify the umbilical anatomy and abdominal wall adiposity. Both extremes of body weight are reasons of extra caution as the obese patient is a challenge for Veress and port insertion entry, while the thin patient, especially the one with an android pelvis and prominent sacral promontory is characterized by an umbilicus lying within 1 or 2 cm of the anterior surface of the aorta.

Technique

a) Induction of general anesthesia
b) palpation of the aortic bifurcation and sacral promontory
c) The abdominal wall should be grasped and elevated between thumb and index finger to ascertain the depth of subcutaneous fat and degree of laxity.

If a palpable pelvic mass extends out of the true pelvis, it should be carefully outlined with a sterile pen while preoperative ultrasound evaluation of visceral adhesions could also be helpful.

Veress Needle

The Veress needle has been designed on purpose to avoid perforation of organs consisting of:

a) a sharp outer cannula
b) a retractable inner cannula with blunt ends.

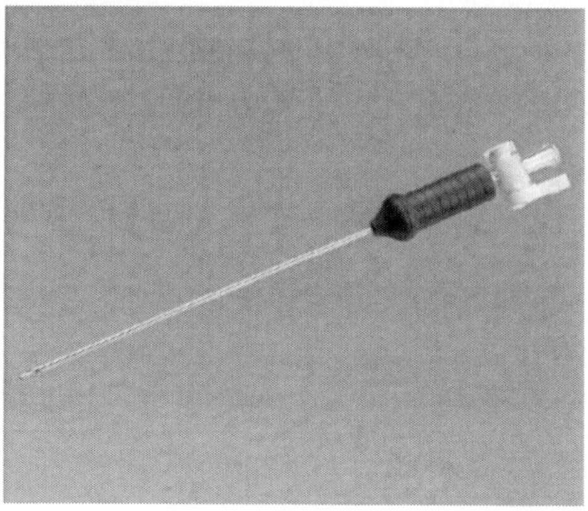

Veress needle.

Steps of insertion

a) Prior to insertion, the anterior abdominal wall is elevated by grasping the wall caudal to the umbilicus with one hand. This maneuver distances the wall from the intra-abdominal contents by 6 to 8cm. If the patient is overweight, two towel clamps can be used on each side of the umbilicus to achieve a similar effect.
b) Sharp entry is best than directly through the base of the umbilicus, which is the thinnest portion of the anterior abdominal wall. The retracted umbilical fossa represents the region of abdominal skin where it is fused to underlying linea alba.
c) The angle of Veress needle insertion should vary accordingly from 45 degrees in non-obese women to 90 degrees in very obese women, but once inserted it should be directed aimed in the midline towards the uterus, away from pelvic blood vessels.
d) When the needle is passing through the abdominal wall, two type of resistance will be felt as it meets and traverses fascia and then peritoneum (two clicks). A distinct click can often be heard as the blunt tip portion of the Veress needle finally springs forward into the peritoneal cavity.
e) During the insertion, tissue resistance compresses an inner spring and a blunt stylet, which is slightly longer than the sharp external needle sheath which retracts, and remains so until the sharp tip of the external needle sheath pierces the peritoneum.
f) When tissue resistance disappears, the blunt cannula is pushed forward by the inner spring to prevent organ or vessel injury.
g) When Veress needle is intra-abdominally, the insufflations of the abdomen with CO2 starts (Gas on).
h) When the intrabdominal pressure is 20 mm Hg, puncture of peritoneum follows with a large trocar.

The most common site of entry is the umbilicus, because it is relatively avascular and the thinnest accessible portion of the anterior abdominal wall. The umbilicus is often located at or cephalad to the aortic bifurcation, and consistently located cephalad to where the left common iliac vein crosses the midline at the sacral promontory.

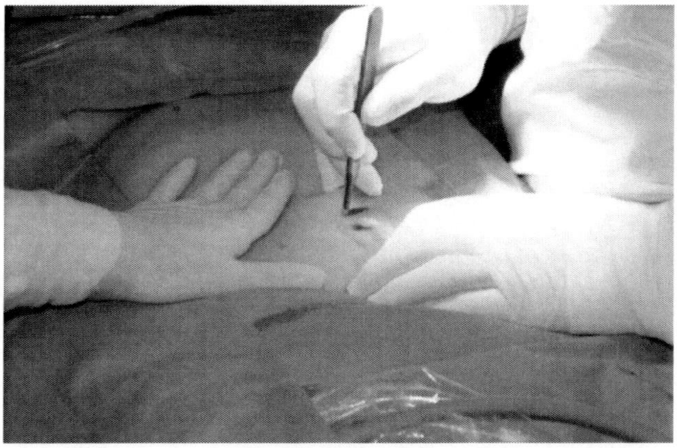

Supraumbilical entry.

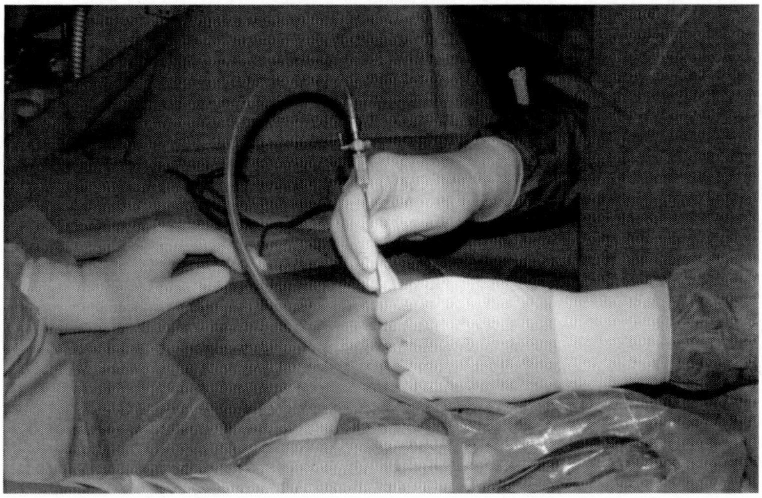

Veress needle entry.

Entry failure of the Veress needle tip leads in the preperitoneal space. For this reason, confirmation of intraabdominal entry prior to gas instillation is necessary and is achieved with:

- a 10-ml syringe filled with 5 ml saline connected to the Veress needle. Free flow of saline into the peritoneal cavity signals peritoneal entry. If saline returns, then preperitoneal placement should be indicated.
- Aspiration is following to clarify if blood is aspirated (vascular injury) and if that happens the needle is left in place and an exploratory laparotomy is following.
- Once the surgeon is certain that the tip of the needle lies within the peritoneal cavity, the abdominal insufflation starts. Observing the actual insufflation pressure to be 8 mm or less and that the gas is flowing freely confirms the intrabdominal entry.

The flow of carbon dioxide should be turned to 1 L/minute, and the indicator on the machine for CO_2 infused should be reset to zero.

If insufflation pressure is high or there is no flow, the Veress should be rotated to assess whether the opening of the needle is resting on the abdominal wall, omentum or bowel or a small piece of tissue is blocking the tip. Veress needle maneuvers in and out should be avoided.

Definitive signs that the Veress needle is intraadominal:

a) loss of dullness to percussion over the liver
b) symmetrical expansion of the abdominal wall
c) An effective system to evaluate sub-umbilical adhesions is to insert a needle connected to a syringe filled with saline solution in the Veress needle. The aspiration of CO_2 confirms the pneumoperitoneum.

Trocar Insertion

When the pressure of pneumoperitoneum reaches 20 mm Hg, the Veress needle is removed and a primary trocar is placed blind in the umbilical incision with an angle of the trocar similar to the Veress needle. The trocar punctures the fascia, and underlying peritoneum and enters the abdominal cavity. A gas rushing sound characteristically confirms placement.

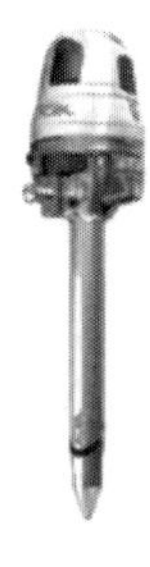

Xcel trocar (Ethicon).

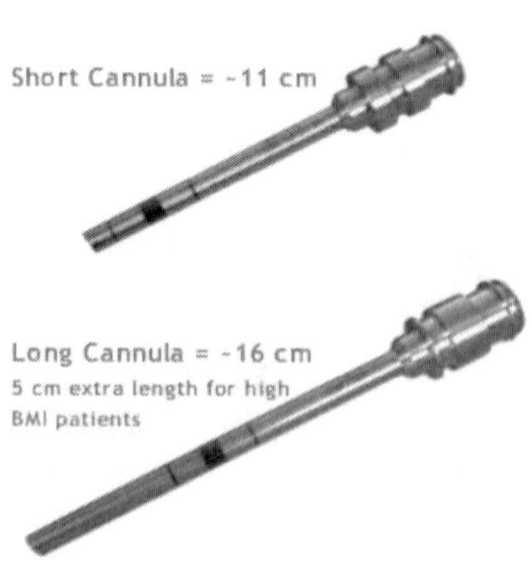

Short and long cannula.

Safety before trocar insertion

- All moveable parts of a reusable trocar should be inspected for tightness and function.
- The spring-loaded mechanism of a disposable-shielded trocar can be checked for proper function by triggering and witnessing engagement through a tracted gauze pad.
- The type of trocar tip affects entry force. For example, force is greater for conical than for pyramidal tips while conical tips theoretically reduce the risk of injury to blood vessels within the abdominal wall. Conical devices penetrate layers of the abdominal wall primarily by dilating rather than cutting.
- A screw-in (turning) technique must be considered when using any trocar with slow steady force.
- The trocar is initially inserted perpendicularly to penetrate the skin and subcutaneous fat. In the non-obese patient, it is then tilted downward at a 60- to 70-degree angle towards the uterus. If the patient is obese, trocar insertion should be completely perpendicular but with controlled minimal entry to ensure the shortest route into the abdominal cavity.
- Increasing pneumoperitoneal pressure to at least 20-mm before trocar insertion further reduces risk by increasing volume, providing firmer countertraction, and pushing peritoneum more firmly against the abdominal wall.
- Optical trocars are visually directed by either a transparent blunt conical tip with plastic tissue separators or a fine, laterally separating blade that provides a sequential view in the monitor of tissues penetrated during insertion as yellow fat, white fascia, red muscle, and transparent peritoneum.

Insertion of Accessory Trocars

a) Trocars are placed using direct laparoscopic visualization to minimize the puncture risk to anterior abdominal wall vessels, bowel, or the bladder.
b) The patient is placed in Trendelenburg position to displace bowel from the pelvis.
c) Care is taken to the superficial epigastric artery which arises from femoral vessels to branch superiorly to supply skin and subcutaneous tissues of the abdominal wall and which can usually be identified by transillumination.
d) A conical tip is less likely to lacerate a vessel than a multiblade pyramidal tip
e) Once the sites are chosen, the skin is incised superficially with a no. 11 blade in Langer's line, just enough to accommodate the diameter of the trocar. A Kelly clamp could be inserted into the subcutaneous defect and the incision is widened enough to allow dissection down to the rectus fascia.
f) The trocar is held so the index or middle finger extends down the sheath to act as a break.
g) The trocar tip is visualized continuously and inserted with a slow motion (side-to-side for pyramidal, twisting for conical, linear for linear cutting) initially in a

perpendicular fashion until it superficially penetrates the fascia. After fascial engagement, the direction of the sheath is directly towards the uterus

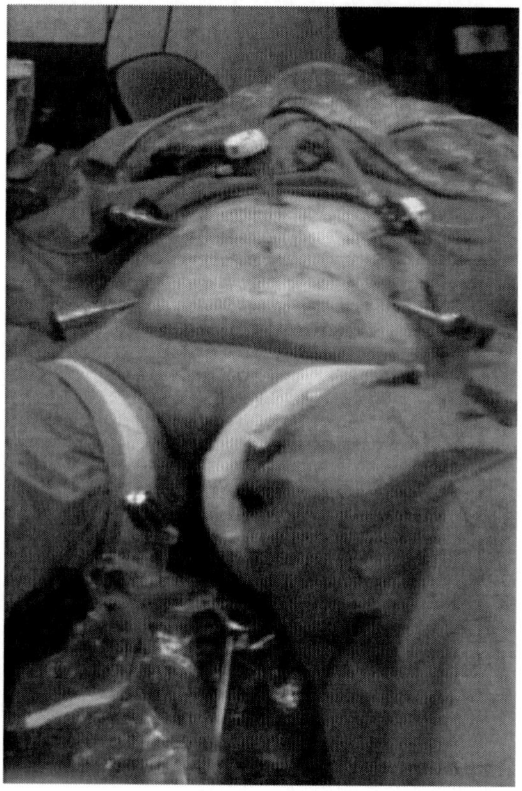

Trocars placement.

Several complications occur during initial insertion of the Veress needle and robotic ports. Vascular and visceral injuries (0.003%-6%) have been reported after veress or ports insertion.

Injury

The most common type of organ injury, during robotic port insertion is bowel injury. Patients with previous laparotomy have a higher incidence of abdominal adhesions. If this complication happens, the patient will present with abdominal pain, fever, nausea and vomiting the first two postoperative days. It was shown that the incidence of bowel injury can reach 0.16%, while 39.8% of vascular and intestinal injuries are caused by the Veress needle, 37.9% by insertion of the primary trocar and 22% by the insertion of the secondary trocar. The major vessels that could be injured during the insertion of either the Veress needle or the trocars include the aorta, vena cava, and common iliac, hypogastric, external iliac, and mesenteric arteries. Bladder injury is a rather rare risk as bladder decompression with catheters and careful placement of secondary trocars under direct vision will prevent the injury.

Chapter 9

The Role of Uterine Manipulators in Robotic Procedures

- the development of minimally invasive surgical techniques (laparoscopic and robotic) has introduced new approaches in the treatment of gynecological cancers
- uterine manipulator is defined as the device that can be applied, through vagina into uterus, during the surgical operation, in order to:
  - facilitate the maneuvers of uterus and
  - assist to clarify the edge of the cervix, particularly in robotic surgery where there is absence of haptic sensation.
  - during the operation an extra member of the surgical team (second assistant) is required either to maintain the instrument in the correct position or to manipulate the uterus according to surgeon's requests. The second assistant has to execute the precise adjustments at the vaginal end and to decide the retraction force applied.
  - The ideal uterine manipulator should be:
    a) safe
    b) easy to fit and utilize
    c) offering a great range of motion of the uterus
    d) cost-effective (either reusable or disposable)

At the moment, a device that combines all the above characteristics does not exist.

Each commercially available manipulator presents distinctive advantages and disadvantages.

We are not presenting all the different types of uterine manipulators, but only the most common used:

Clermond-Ferrand uterine manipulator

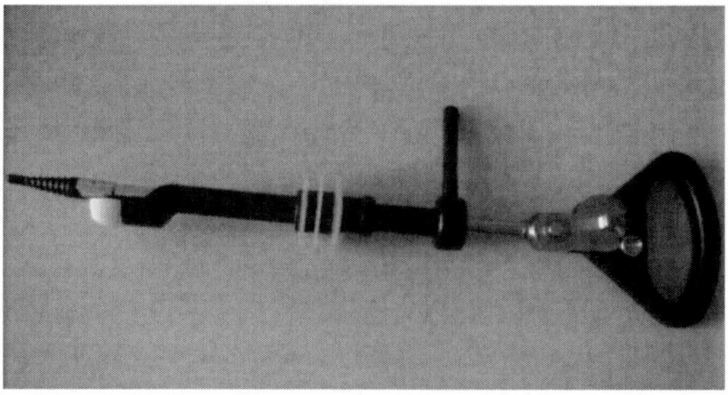

Clermond-Ferrand uterine manipulator.

Pro:

- movement ranges +140° in the anterior plane, +90° in the posterior plane
- permits independent movements
- permits easy grasping of the uterine pedicles and lateral fornices
- reusable
- pneumoperitoneum can be easily maintained

Cons:

- necessitates dilatation of the cervix
- complex to assemble
- expensive instrument

Hohl Uterine Manipulator

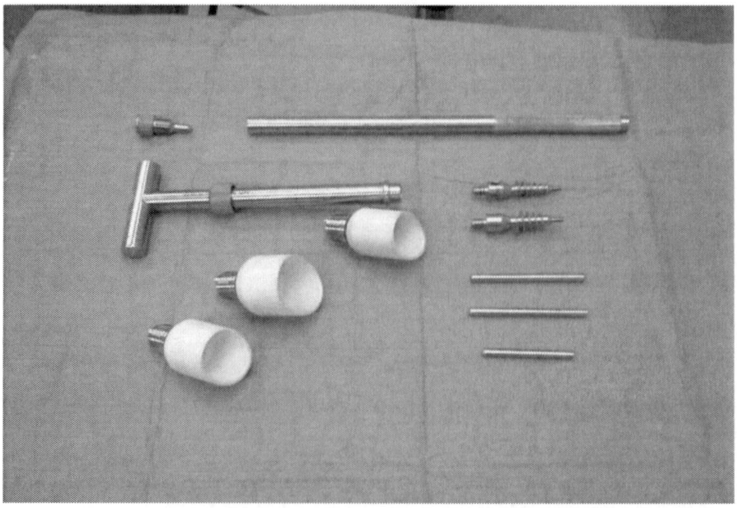

Hohl Uterine Manipulator.

Pro:

- movement ranges +130° in the anterior plane, +90° in the posterior plane
- permits independent movements
- reusable
- pneumoperitoneum can be easily maintained

Cons:

- elevation of the uterus is limited
- effective only in hysterectomy procedures
- the initial fixation of the device can cause bleeding from the cervix

Clearview or Endopath® Uterine Manipulator

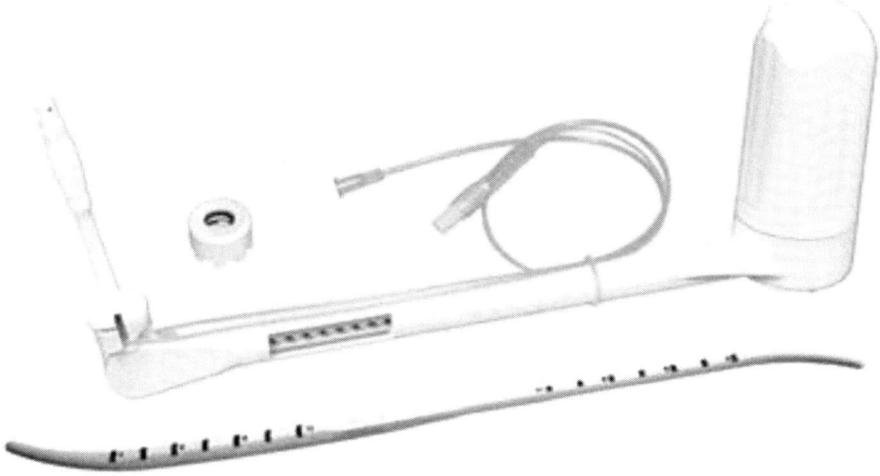

Endopath® Uterine Manipulator.

Pro:

- movement ranges +130° in the anterior plane, +90° in the posterior plane

Cons:

- does not present easily the vaginal fornices
- not reusable
- pneumoperitoneum can be maintained with difficulty

RUMI® uterine manipulator with Koh colpotomizer™

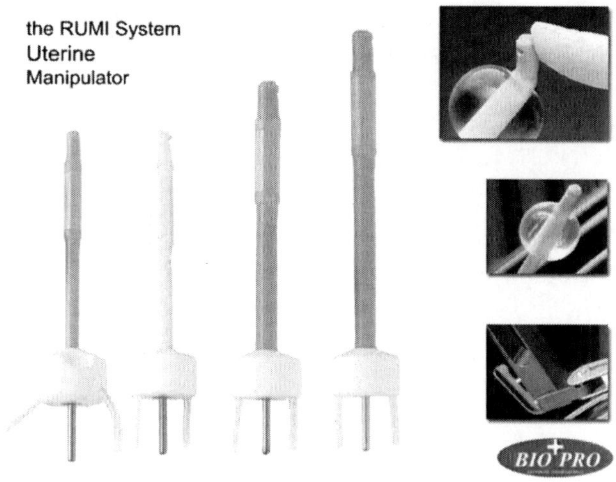

The RUMI system (Continued).

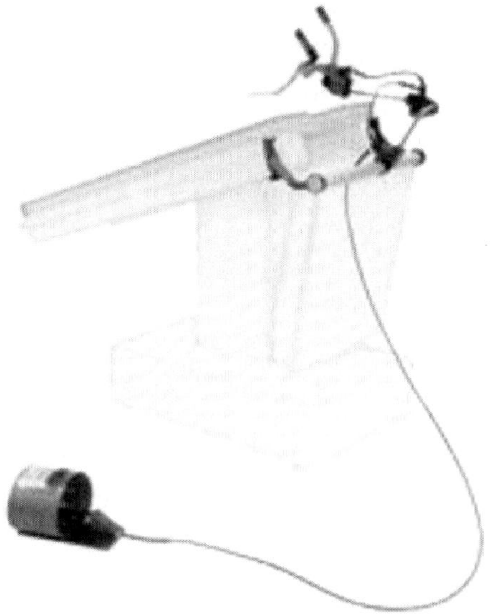

The RUMI system.

Pro:

- the tip of the device can rotate 140°
- pneumoperitoneum can be easily maintained
- can be used with both with harmonic and ultrasonic coagulating shears

Cons:

- elevation of the uterus is limited

- complex to assemble
- partially reusable

Hourcabie Uterine Manipulator

Pro:

- permits easy grasping of the uterine pedicles and lateral fornices with automatic staplers
- independent movement of the manipulator shaft
- reusable
- easy to assemble

Cons:

- restricted range of uterine movements
- pneumoperitoneum can be maintained with difficulty

V-Care® Uterine Manipulator

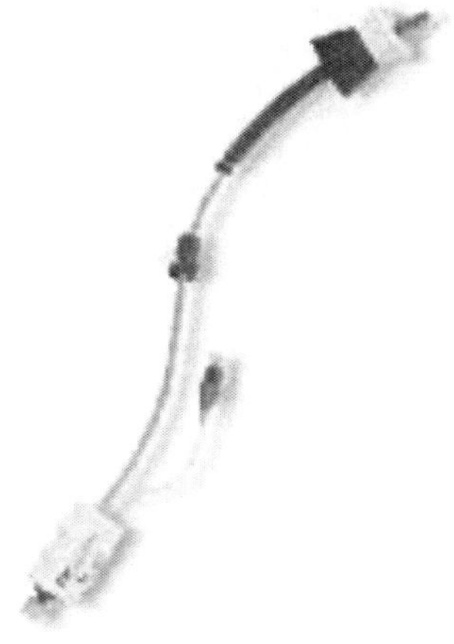

V care uterine manipulator.

Pro:

- permits a great range of uterine movements
- good presentation of the vaginal fornices
- permits independent movements
- pneumoperitoneum can be easily maintained
- easy manipulation

Cons:

- not reusable
- can not be used with laser shears
- the manipulation of large uteri is difficult

Total laparoscopic hysterectomy (TLH)-Dr Mangeshikar® uterine manipulator

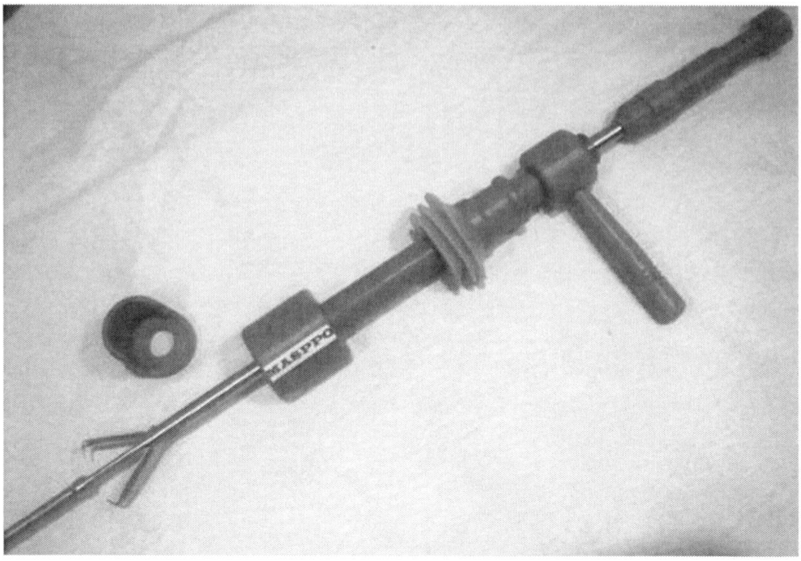

Mangeshikar uterine manipulator.

Mangeshikar® uterine manipulator

Pro:

- movement ranges +130° in the anterior plane, +90° in the posterior plane
- good presentation of the vaginal fornices
- reusable
- pneumoperitoneum can be easily maintained

Cons:

- limited uterine manipulation

McCartney Tube

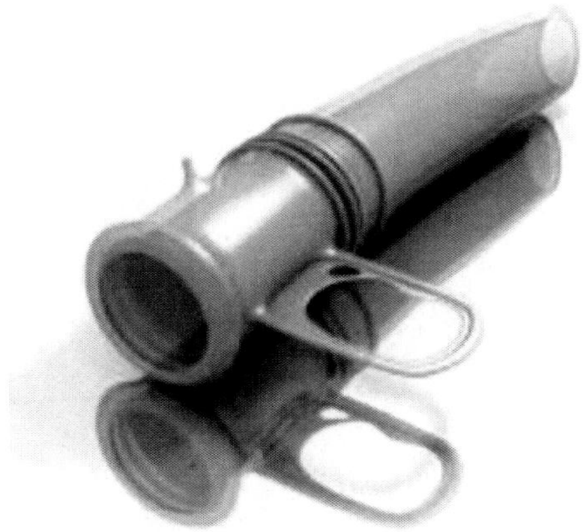

McCartney Tube.

Pro:

- reduces tumour seeded contamination risks during removal
- the soft curvature acts as a safe guide during sectioning of the uterus and ensures no trauma to the tissue
- the airtight valves prevent loss of pneumoperitoneum after colpotomy.

Cons:

- not reusable
- the manipulation of large uteri is difficult

Chapter 10

Pelvic Anatomy

Abdominal Wall

The musculature of the abdominal wall is composed of 2 muscle groups:

a) the flat muscles (external oblique, internal oblique, and the transversus abdominis)
b) the second group which run vertically, the rectus abdominis and the pyramidalis

More analytically:

i. The external oblique muscle is the largest and most superficial of the flat muscles of the abdominal wall. Arising from the lower 8 ribs, the external oblique courses transversely to insert upon the iliac crests. The aponeurosis is a strong tendinous sheath that ends medially in the linea alba.

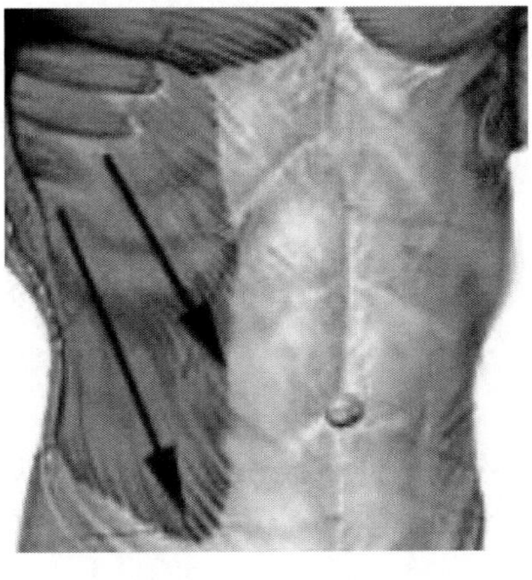

External oblique muscle.

ii. The internal oblique muscle arises from the upper surface of the inguinal ligament, the iliac crest, and the thoracolumbar fascia. This muscle courses at a right angle to the fibers of the external oblique muscle. The aponeurosis of the internal oblique splits at the edge of the rectus muscle to envelope the rectus. The anterior layer blends with the aponeurosis of the external oblique. Posterior to the rectus muscle, this aponeurosis blends with the aponeurosis of the transversus abdominis to form a portion of the posterior rectus sheath.

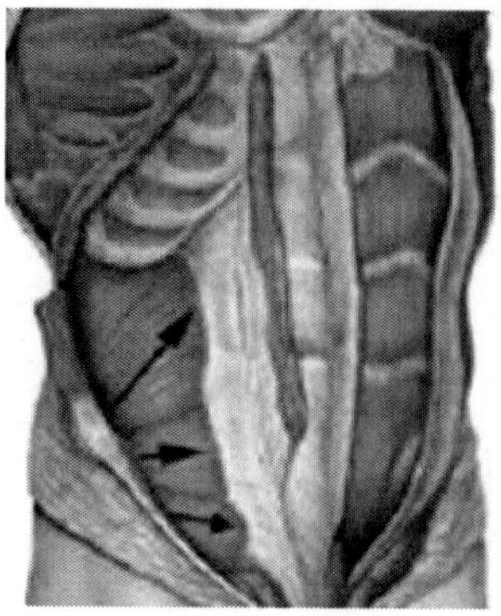

Internal oblique muscle.

iii. The transversus abdominis muscle arises from the inguinal ligament, the iliac crest, the thoracolumbar fascia, and the lower costal cartilages. Coursing transversely to the midline, the upper three fourths of the transversus aponeurosis lies behind the rectus muscle. The lower one fourth of the aponeurosis passes in front of the rectus muscle. The aponeurosis of each flat muscle joins medial to the rectus muscle to form the linea alba.

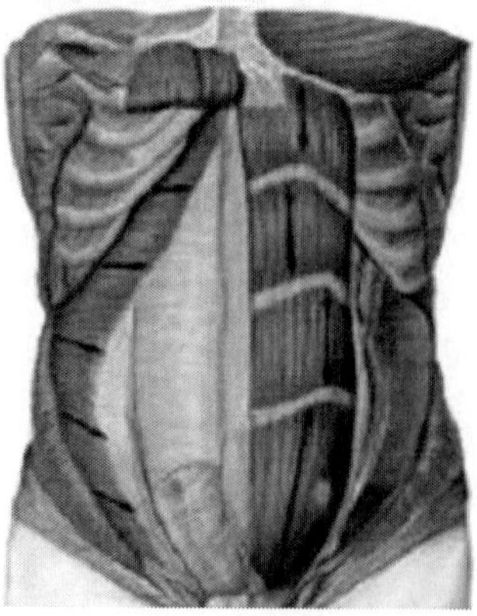

Transversus abdominis muscle.

iv. The rectus muscle runs vertically to insert into the xiphoid process and the fifth, sixth, and seventh costal cartilages. The muscle fibers contain 3 fibrous insertions known as the linea transversae. The rectus is surrounded by the rectus sheath, which consists of the aponeuroses of the oblique muscles and the transversus abdominis. A small, vestigial, triangular-shaped muscle, the pyramidalis, arises from the symphysis and inserts upon the linea alba. This muscle marks the midline and assists in the identification of the medial borders of the rectus muscle.

Important Surgical Landmarks

a) The linea alba is in the midline between the 2 rectus muscles. Formed by the fusion of the aponeuroses of the external oblique, internal oblique, and transversus abdominis, identifying this structure during a midline incision is important.
b) The arcuate line that is found below the rectus muscle, approximately halfway between the umbilicus and the symphysis pubis. Above the arcuate line, the aponeuroses of the internal oblique and transversus abdominis fuse to form the posterior rectus sheath. Below the arcuate line, the posterior rectus sheath is absent.

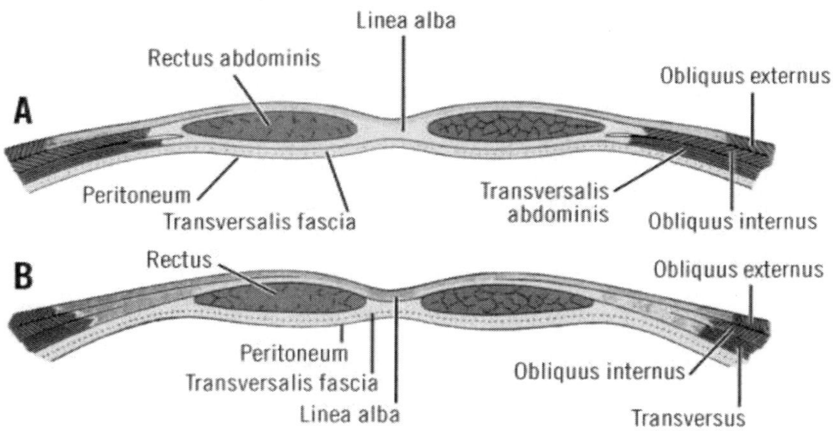

Surgical landmarks.

Blood Supply

The primary blood supply to the abdominal wall is from the superficial and deep vasculature.

The superficial vasculature originates from branches of the femoral artery and includes the superficial epigastric, the superficial circumflex, and the superficial external pudendal arteries. These vessels course through the tissues anterior to the rectus sheath.

The deep vasculature is composed of vessels from the external iliac artery and the internal thoracic artery. The inferior epigastric artery originates from the external iliac artery and courses posterior to the lateral one third of the rectus muscle. Another branch of the external iliac is the deep circumflex artery, which courses cephalad lateral to the inferior epigastric artery. The superior epigastric artery is the terminal branch of the internal thoracic artery. This artery has multiple branches leading to the rectus muscle and has an anastomosis with the inferior epigastric artery. The internal thoracic artery is the source of the musculophrenic artery, which has an anastomosis with the deep circumflex artery.

Inferior Epigastric Vessels

- Originate from the external iliac vessels before entry beneath the inguinal ligament
- Courses medial to the round ligament
- Travels underneath the lateral third of the rectus abdominis muscles
- Typically not visualized by transillumination

Superficial Epigastric Vessels

- Courses within the subcutaneous tissue of the anterior abdominal wall
- May be visualized by transillumination
- Follows a similar course to the inferior epigastric vessels

Uterine arteries provide the principal blood supply to the female internal genital organs. These arteries are branches from the internal iliac (hypogastric) arteries.

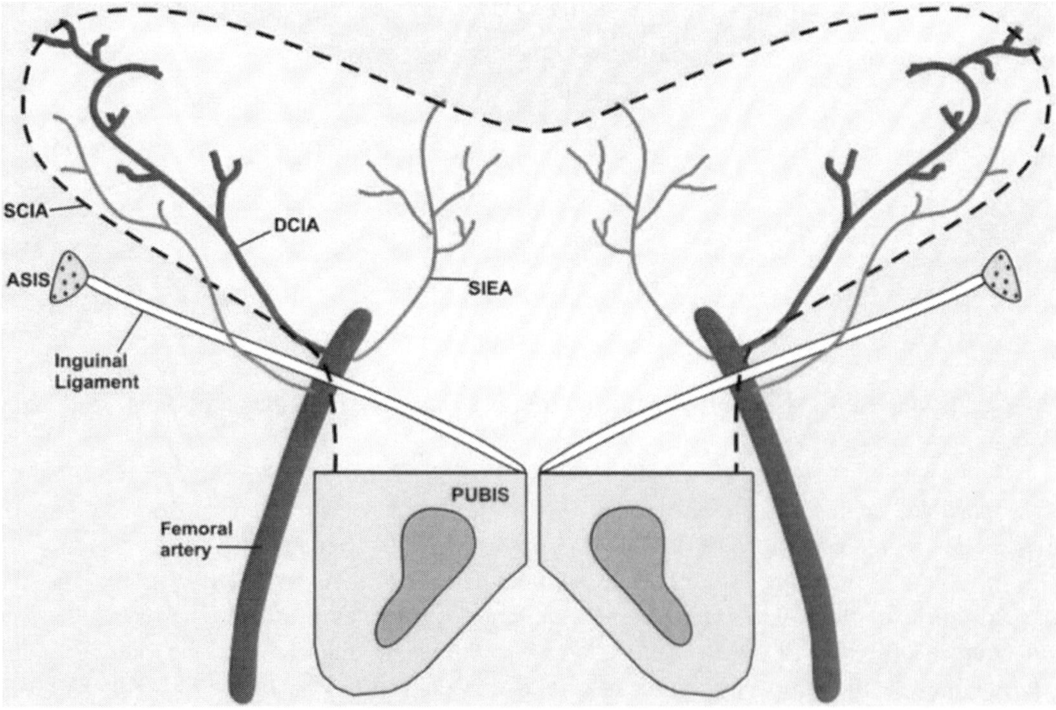

ASIS-anterior superior iliac spine; SCIA-superficial circumflex iliac artery; DCIA-deep circumflex iliac artery; SIEA-superficial inferior epigastric artery.

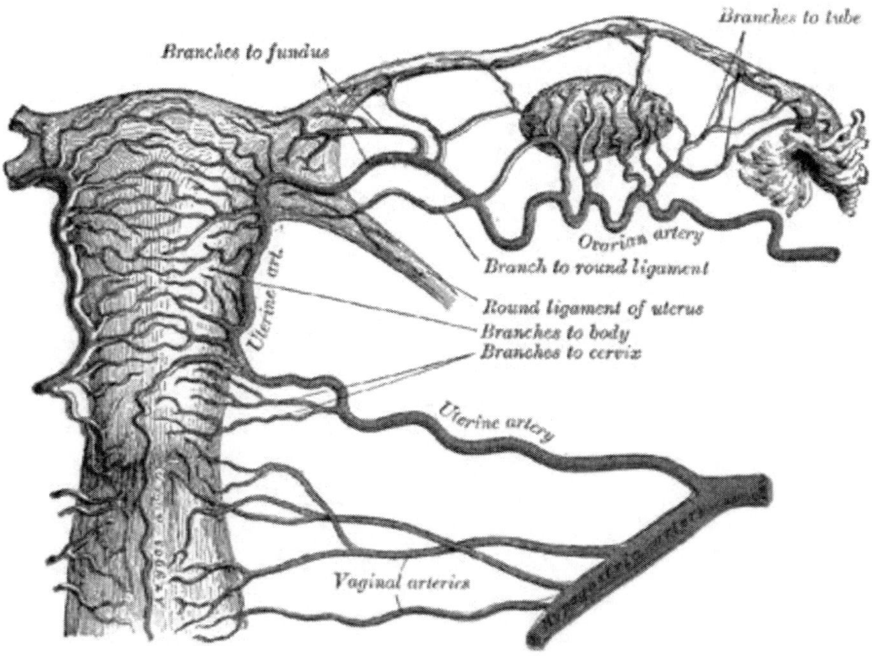

Arteries of the female genital tract.

The uterine artery runs medially above the cardinal ligament and crosses anterior to the ureter en route to the cervix. The artery forms extensive vascular networks lateral to the vagina, the fallopian tube, the uterine fundus, and the ovary. The vagina is also supplied by vaginal arteries that take origin from the internal iliac arteries.

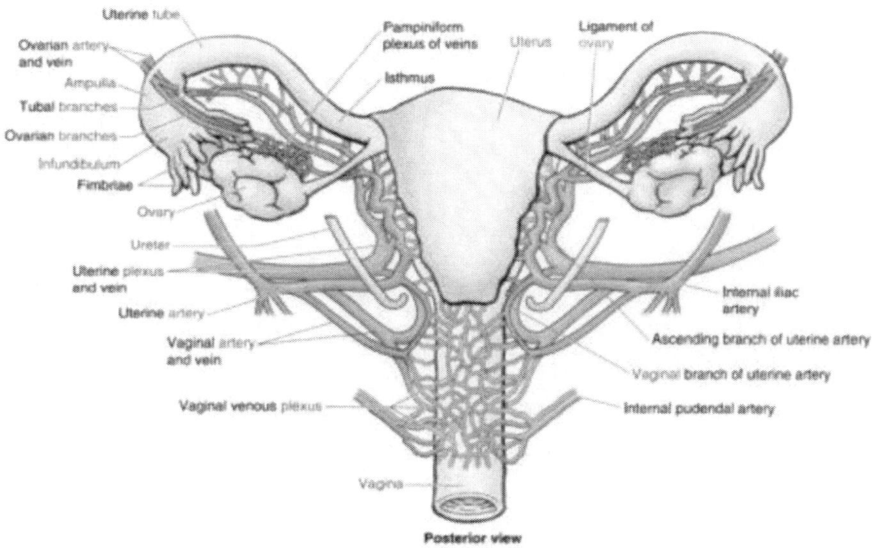

Vessels of the female genital tract.

The venous drainage of the upper part of vagina, cervix, uterus as well as ovaries is performed through a wide plexus of small veins that are located between the layers of the broad ligament. This plexus forms veins that mainly run in parallel with the arterial blood supply.

Nerve Supply

Innervation by:

- the thoracoabdominal nerve
- the ilioinguinal nerve
- the iliohypogastric nerve

The thoracoabdominal nerve travels caudad between the transversus abdominis and the internal oblique. This nerve innervates the flat muscles of the abdominal wall and the rectus muscle. Innervating the lower abdominal wall are the iliohypogastric nerve and the ilioinguinal nerve. Both of these nerves arise primarily from the first lumbar nerve root. Damage to these nerves results in sensory changes in the mons pubis and the labium major.

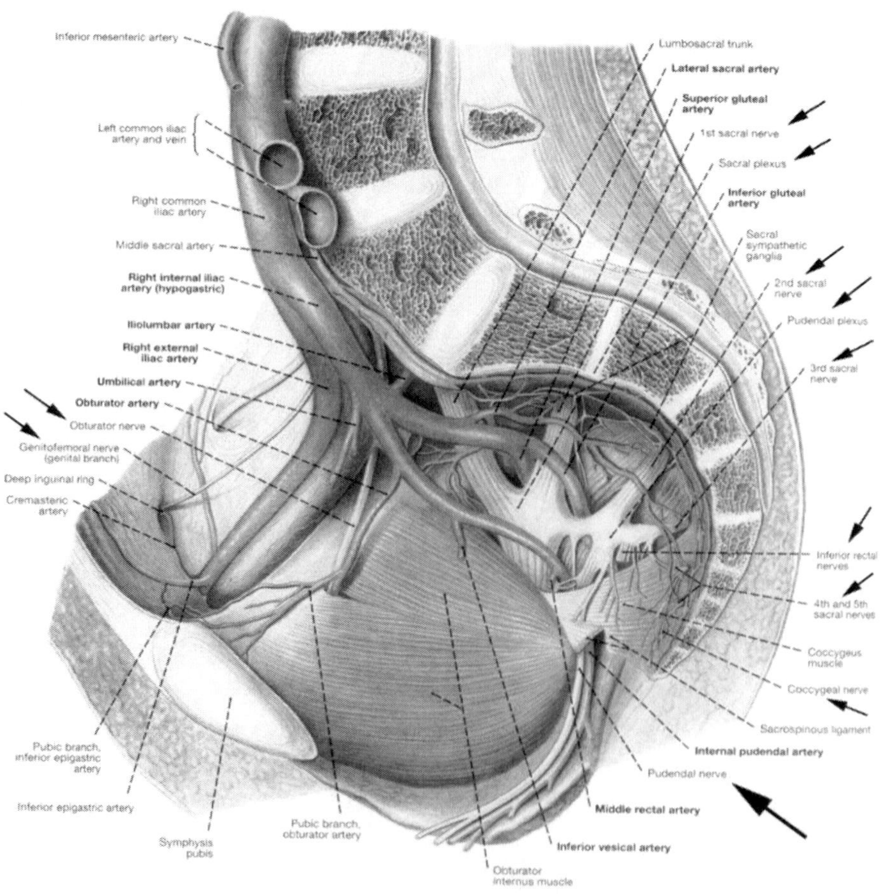

Nerves and vessels of the pelvis.

The iliohypogastric nerve is a branch of the first lumbar nerve. It runs through the upper part of the lateral border of the psoas major. Then, it passes down and laterally across the quadratus lumborum muscle behind the kidney to the crest of the ilium. There it passes through the transversus abdominis muscle. Then it divides into a lateral cutaneous and a anterior cutaneous branch. The first passes between the internal and external oblique muscles, and supplies the skin over the gluteal region. The anterior cutaneous branch runs along the crest of the ilium, and through the internal oblique muscle, passes the aponeurosis of the external oblique muscle almost two centimeters above the external superficial inguinal ring. It innervates the rectus abdominis and pyramidalis, while part of iliohypogastric nerve also the skin over the hypogastrium and the posterolateral gluteal region.

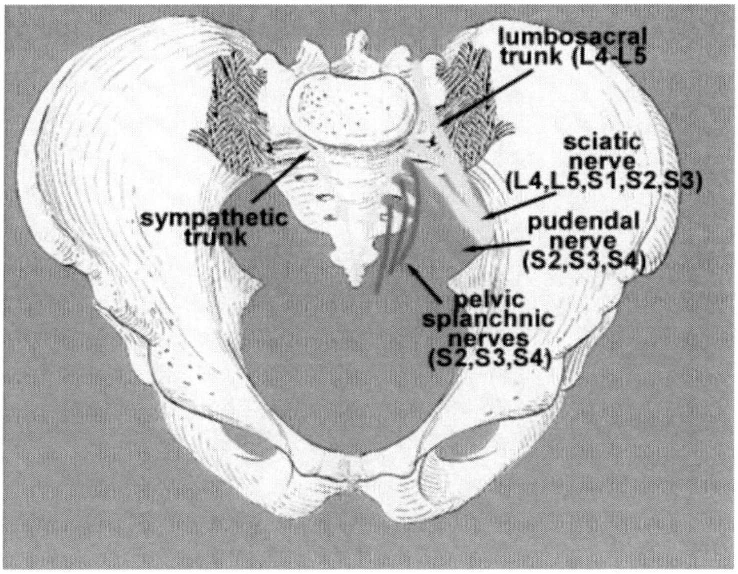

Nerves in the pelvis.

The ilioinguinal nerve also takes origin from a branch of the first lumbar nerve (L1). It runs on the lateral border of the psoas major and passes obliquely across the quadratus lumborum muscle. The ilioinguinal nerve through the transversus abdominis meets with the iliohypogastric nerve between the transversus and the internal oblique muscle. The two nerves run together through the superficial inguinal ring. Fibers of ilioinguinal nerve are distributed to the skin of the upper and medial part of the thigh, and to the skin covering the mons pubis and labium majus.

Landmarks of the anterior abdominal wall
- Umbilicus
- Anterior superior iliac spines
- Pubic symphysis

Superficial pelvic and peritoneal structures
– Median umbilical fold
- Peritoneal covering of the median umbilical ligament/urachus

– Medial umbilical folds

- Peritoneal covering of the obliterated umbilical arteries
- Allow laparoscopic surgeon to identify uterine artery because of origin from internal iliac artery

– Lateral umbilical folds

- Peritoneal covering of the inferior epigastric vessels
- Direct hernias occurs medial to the lateral umbilical fold
- Indirect hernias originates lateral to the umbilical fold
- Hasselbach's Triangle:
  a) Laterally: Inferior Epigastrics artery and vein_
  b) Medially: Rectus Sheath
  c) Inferiorly: Inguinal Ligament
  d) Posteriorly: Transversalis Fascia

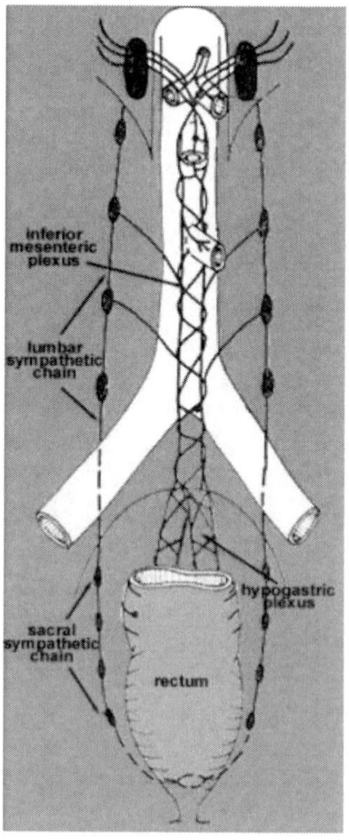

Nerve plexuses.

Urachus

- Courses from the bladder to the umbilicus in the midline beneath the anterior abdominal wall and median umbilical fold
- Lies in the space of Retzius, between the transversalis fascia anteriorly and the peritoneum posteriorly
- Lumen normally becomes obliterated during embryonic development, thus becoming a functionless remnant
- Patent urachus is rare

Ureters

- Enter pelvic cavity at the pelvic brim
- Course superficial to the common iliac artery and deep to the infundibulopelvic ligament
- Travel in the medial leaf of the broad ligament
- Pass lateral to the uterosacral ligament and beneath the uterine artery lateral to the cervix
- Travel in an endopelvic fascia tunnel medially and anteriorly along the upper part of the vagina, and enter into the bladder wall and then open into the trigone

Pelvic Blood Supply

- Aorta
  - Middle sacral artery
- Common iliac artery
- External iliac artery
  - Inferior epigastric artery
  - Deep circumflex iliac artery
- Posterior division of internal iliac artery
  - Superior gluteal artery
  - Iliolumbar artery
  - Lateral sacral
- Anterior division of internal iliac artery
  - Obturator artery
  - Uterine artery
  - Superior vesical artery
  - Inferior vesical artery
  - Umbilical ligament
  - Middle rectal artery
  - Internal pudendal artery
- Inferior rectal artery
- Labial arteries
- Dorsal artery of the clitoris

The internal iliac artery is the major artery of the pelvis. It supplies the walls and viscera of the pelvis, the majority of the pelvic organs and the medial compartment of the thigh. The internal iliac artery derives from the bifurcation of the common iliac artery, at the lumbosacral articulation, while is running downward to the upper margin of the greater sciatic foramen, splits into two large branches, the anterior and the posterior. Generally, there is great variability in the exact arrangement of branches of the internal iliac artery.

The external iliac artery derives by the bifurcation of the common iliac artery, anterior to the sacroiliac joint. It provides the main blood supply to the legs. It runs downwards, along the brim of the pelvis and splits in two large branches - the inferior epigastric artery and the deep circumflex artery. These branches provide blood to the muscles and skin in the lower abdominal wall. The external iliac artery after passes under the inguinal ligament becomes the femoral artery.

Pelvic Nerves

a. Femoral nerve

– Nerve roots L2, L3, L4
– Provides motor function to the extensor muscles
– Provides sensation to the thigh

b. Sciatic nerve

– Nerve roots L4, L5, S1, S2, S3
– Largest nerve in the body
– It divides into the tibial and peroneal nerves
– Provides motor function to the distal extremity

c. Obturator nerve

– Nerve roots L2, L3, L4
– Provides motor function to the adductor muscles

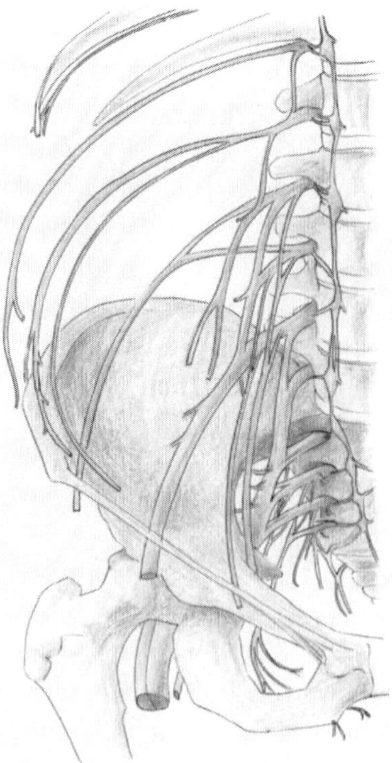

Nerve roots.

The obturator nerve originates from the roots L2, L3 and L4 nerves. It passes through psoas major muscle and from its medial side close to the brim of the pelvis goes behind the common iliac arteries, while passes along the lateral wall of the lesser pelvis, and through the obturator canal enters the thigh. At the thigh, it splits into two branches, an anterior and a posterior. The obturator nerve innervates the skin of the medial aspect of the thigh while also provides motor function to the adductor muscles.

d. Pudendal nerve

- Nerve roots S2, S3, S4
- Provides motor functions to the muscles of the pelvis and extern al anal sphincter
- Provides sensation to the vulva and clitoris

e. Genitofemoral nerve

- Nerve roots L1, L2
- Provides sensation to the thigh and vulva

The genitofemoral nerve takes origin from the L1-L2 segments of the lumbar plexus. It directs downwards to the anterior surface of the psoas major muscle. The nerve divides into two branches, the genital and the femoral branch. The first (genital) branch passes through the internal inguinal ring, entering in the inguinal canal. Through the inguinal canal, in men, the genital branch provides sensation to the scrotal skin while in women, follows the round ligament of uterus, innervating the skin of the mons pubis and labia majora. The femoral branch goes under the inguinal ligament, following the external iliac artery, provides sensation at the skin of the upper, anterior thigh.

Muscles of the Pelvis

a. Psoas
   - L2, L3, L4 flexes thigh

b. Piriformis
   - S1, S2 rotates thigh laterally

c. Obturator internus
   - L5, S1, S2 rotates thigh laterally

d. Levator Ani
   - Pubococcygeus S3, S4 raise pelvic floor
   - Iliococcygeus
   - Puborectalis

e. Coccygeus
   - S4, S5 raise pelvic floor

Bladder

- Muscular structure which functions as a reservoir for urine
- Can hold 1000 ml however most females have a strong urge to void at 400 ml
- Supplied by the superior vesical and inferior vesical arteries
- Innervation is both parasympathetic and sympathetic
- Parasympathetic (S2, S3, S4) controls detrusor contraction while inhibiting the internal sphincter
- Sympathetic (T11, T12, L1, L2) transmit sensation

Rectum

- Last portion of the colon, rich blood supply, relatively mobile below the peritoneum
- Multiple layers which control continence
  - 1st it follows the contour of the sacrum
  - 2nd the valves of houston produce sharp turns for the feces to navigate
  - 3rd the puborectalis muscles forms a sling around the rectum called the anorectal angle
  - All these layers close off the lumen with valsalva
- The pectinate line marks the transformation from squamous epithelium to columnar epithelium
- Blood supply stems from both the IMA and the internal iliac arteries (superior, middle, inferior rectal arteries)

Pelvic Group of Lymph Nodes

The lymph nodes of the pelvis can be divided into parietal, which lying behind the peritoneum and in close association with the larger blood vessels; and in visceral, which are found in relation to the visceral arteries.

Parietal nodes of the pelvis

Common Iliac Lymph Nodes

Medial common iliac
Intermediate common iliac
Lateral common iliac
Subaortic common iliac
Common iliac nodes of promontory

External Iliac Lymph Nodes

Medial external iliac

Intermediate external iliac
Lateral external iliac
Medial lacunar (femoral)
Intermediate lacunar (femoral)
Lateral lacunar (femoral)
Interiliac external iliac
Obturator (external iliac obturatory)

Lymph nodes (visceral) of the pelvis

Internal Iliac Lymph Nodes (hypogastric)

Superior gluteal
Interior gluteal
Sacral

Perivesicular Lymph Nodes

Prevesicular
Paravaginal Lymph Nodes
Lateral vesicular
Parauterine Lymph Nodes

Paraaortic Group of Lymph Nodes

The paraaortic lymph nodes are situated at the front of the lumbar vertebral bodies in close proximity to the aorta. These particular lymph nodes drain the upper gastrointestinal tract as well as the abdominal organs.

Paraaortic lymph nodes are divided into three subgroups:

- Preaortic: receive drainage from the part of the gastrointestinal tract, situated above the mid-rectum.
- Retroaortic: receive drainage from the lateral and preaortic lymph nodes.
- Lateral: receive drainage from the iliac lymph nodes and many pelvic organs.

Chapter 11

Gynaecological Robotic Procedures (Indications and Contraindications)

Classification

Level 1

Diagnostic laparoscopy
Sterilisation
Aspiration of ovarian cyst
Ovarian biopsy

Level 2

Division of filmy adhesions
Linear salpingotomy or salpingectomy for ectopic pregnancy
Salpingostomy for infertility
Ovarian cystectomy
Treatment of endometrioma
Salpingo-oophorectomy
Ovarian drilling with laser or diathermy for polycystic ovaries
Treatment of AFS Stage I and II endometriosis
Myomectomy for pedunculated subserous fibroid
Uterosacral nerve ablation
Robotic simple hysterectomy without significant pathology

Level 3

Division of thick adhesions
Robotic radical hysterectomy
Myomectomy for intramural fibroids
Treatment of AFS Stage III and IV endometriosis

Pelvic and para-aortic lymphadenectomy
Pelvic side wall and ureteric dissection
Presacral neurectomy
Incontinence procedures
Prolapse procedures

Advantages of Robotic Applications in Gynaecology

Hysterectomy

rarely conversions to laparotomy
overall operative time: 122.9 minutes
mean estimated blood loss: 79 mL
mean length of hospital stay: 1 day
uterine weight>250 g results in a significantly longer operative time

Reproductive Surgery

Myomectomy
less postoperative morbidity
faster recovery
removal of a mean of 1.6 myomas with a diameter of 7.9 cm
No blood transfusions
conversion to laparotomy: 8.6%
reduced length of stay

Tubal Anastomosis

visualization of a very small diameter lumen and precise suturing with fine-gauge material
longer operative times
shorter hospitalization time and recovery
equal tubal patency and postprocedure pregnancy rates

Reconstructive Pelvic Surgery

sacrocolpopexy,
less blood loss
longer total operative time
shorter length of stay

higher incidence of postoperative fever
low complication rate
low morbidity
fistula repair
meticulous dissection and suturing required to complete this operation laparoscopically is greatly afforded by the robot
uneventful recovery

Gynaecological Oncology

radical hysterectomy for cervical cancer
Median operative time: 3.5 hours
Median blood loss: 300 mL
No complications
Hospital stay: 1 day
mean number of lymph nodes resected does not differ
robotic-assisted hysterectomy with staging for endometrial cancer
conversion rate to laparotomy: 6.7%
low intraoperative and postoperative complications
<10 cases to achieve proficiency

General Advantages

Dexterity
Flexibility
Well-developed technology
Proved efficacy
3D visualization
Increased degrees of motion
Elimination of tremor
Good geometric accuracy
Surgeon comfort

Disadvantages

Cost
Loss of haptics
Requires additional training and time
Larger trocar size compared with laparoscopy

Contraindications

Absolute:

- Severe cardiac disease (Class IV) may not tolerate the deep Trendelenburg positions
- Intestinal obstruction with distended bowel

Relative:

- Multiple previous major surgeries
- Morbid obesity
- Pregnancy beyond five months gestation must be approached with a great deal of caution
- Severe, chronically ill patients

Chapter 12

Fibroids

Definition:

- Tumors situated in uterine myometrium, of unknown aetiology. They are devided as subserosal, intramural, submucosal, pedunctulated.

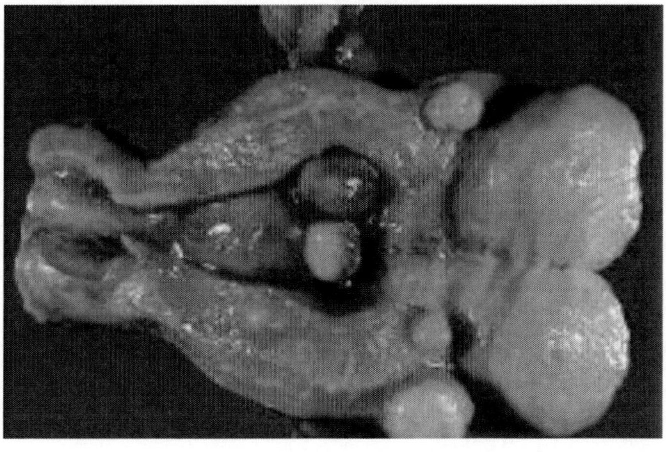

Fibroid uterus.

Incidence:

- >20% of Caucasian women over 30 years old.

Symptoms:

- mainly asymptomatic
- menorrhagia
- abdominal distension (in case of large dimensions fibroids)
- pain (in case of torsion or fibroid degeneration)

Diagnosis:

- abdominal examination (in case of large dimensions)
- ultrasonography
- hysteroscopy
- endometrial biopsy

Medical management:

- oral contraceptive therapy (relieves uterine bleeding and abdominal cramps)
- progesterons, gestrinone, danazol, ulipristal acetate, levonorgestrel intrauterine devices and GnRH analogues could relieve the symptoms

Surgical management:

- surgical treatment (myomectomy) is advised when medical management is not successful for women who want to preserve uterus.
- uterine artery embolization
- radio frequency ablation
- uterine artery ligation
- myomectomy
- hysterectomy

Surgical Steps for Robotic Management

Robotic Myomectomy

Candidates for robotic myomectomy: patients with any single fibroid<15 cm or with < 15 fibroids in total.

Non candidates: patients with a uterine fundus that is palpable above the umbilicus, with diffuse adenomyosis or whose uterine cavity cannot be clearly visualized by imaging techniques

Assessment

Preoperative MRI is used to determine fibroid size, number, and locations, and to rule out adenomyosis.

Basic Setup

Patient in dorsal lithotomy position in Allen stirrups with the arms padded and tucked. After trocar placement, the patient is located in Trendelenburg position. Side-docking is preferred.

The assistant's laparoscopic port is used for suction/irrigation, passage of needles, tissue retraction, and morcellation.

Preferred robotic instruments: the Maryland bipolar forceps, harmonic shears, and Mega needle driver

Technique

- fibroid location exactly determined

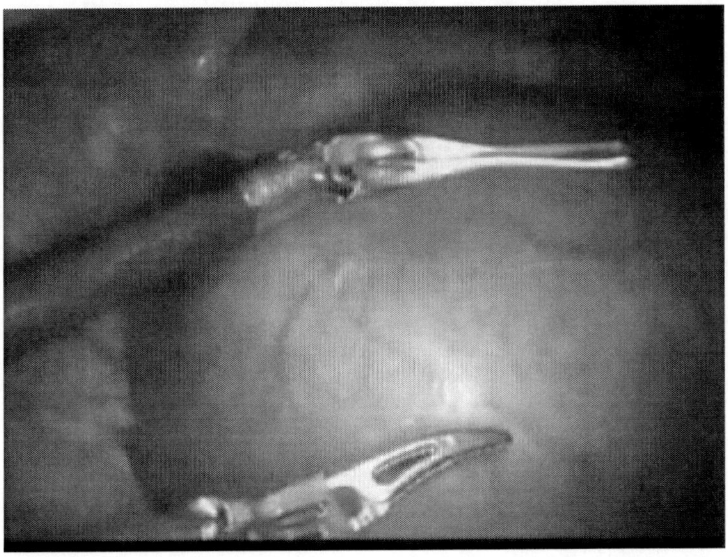

Fibroid location.

- a dilute concentration of vasopressin is injected into the myometrium surrounding the fibroid

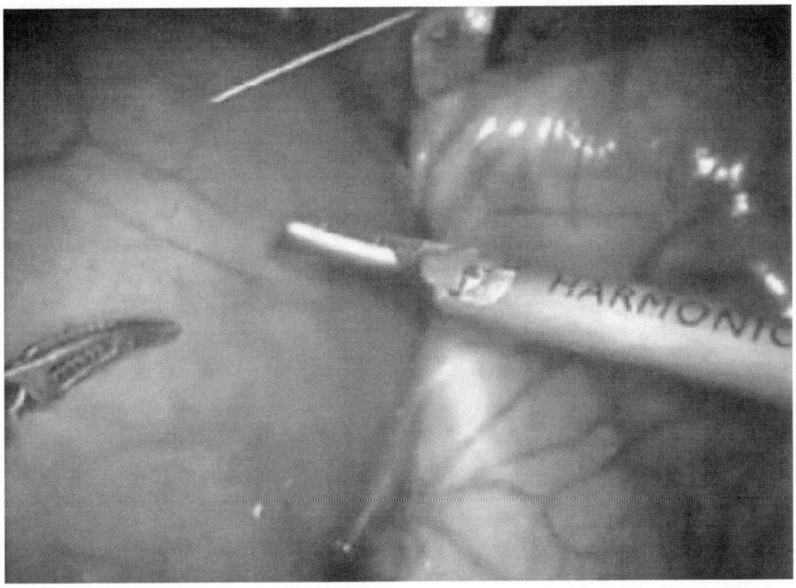

Vasopressin injection.

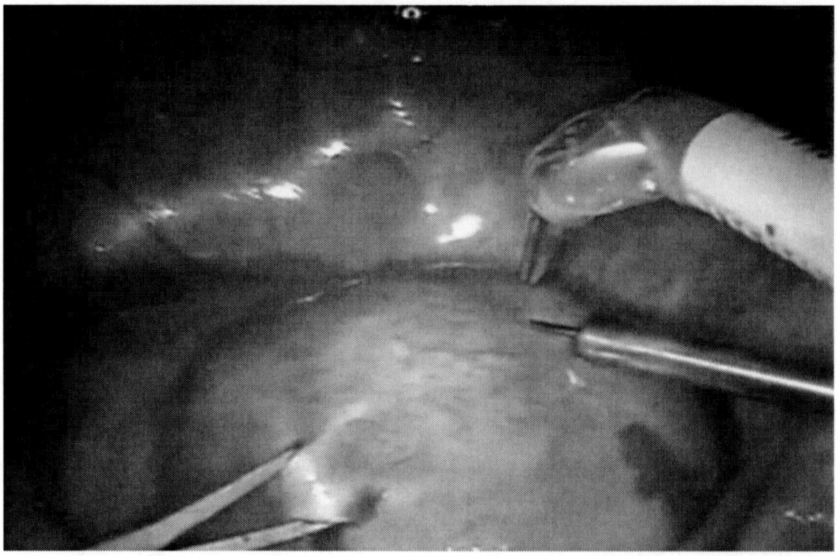

Vasopressin injection.

- hysterotomy is made over the fibroid in a longitudinal or horizontal axis

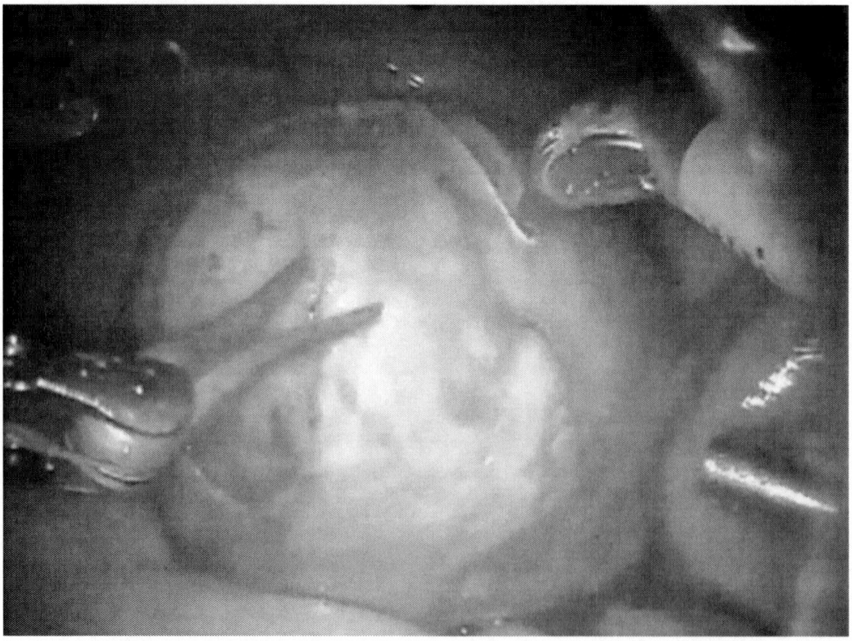

Hysterotomy.

- enucleation of the fibroid by using a robotic tenaculum and/or a bipolar coagulator in addition to the harmonic shears

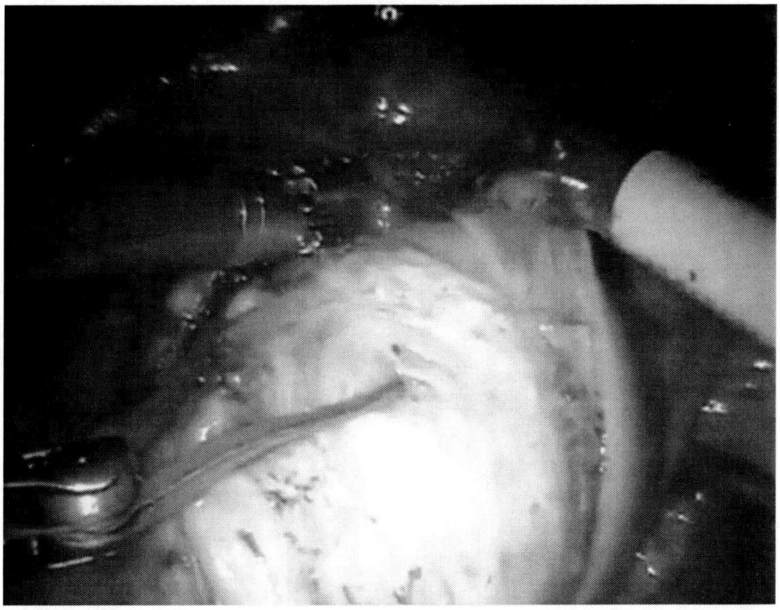

Fibroid enucleation.

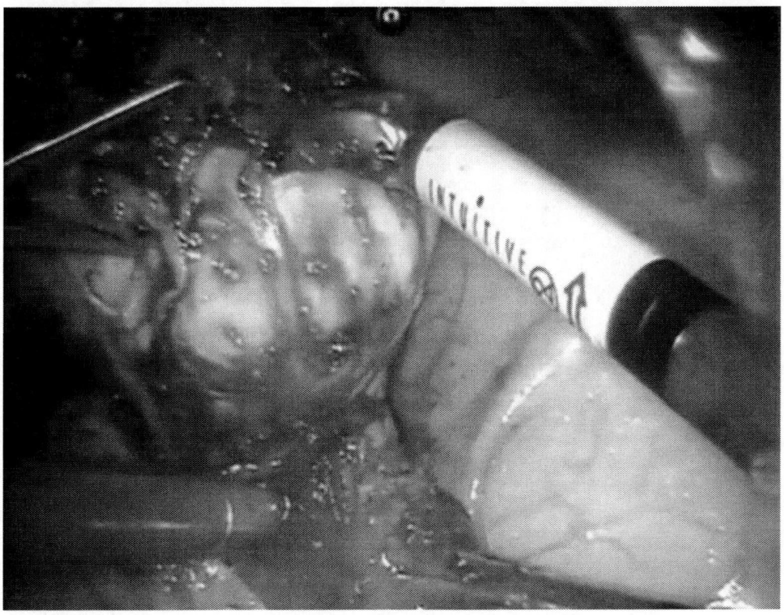

Fibroid enucleation.

- additional traction by the assistant on the fibroid using a laparoscopic tenaculum might be necessary
- hysterotomy multilayer closure employing sutures and suturing techniques similar to those of an open myomectomy

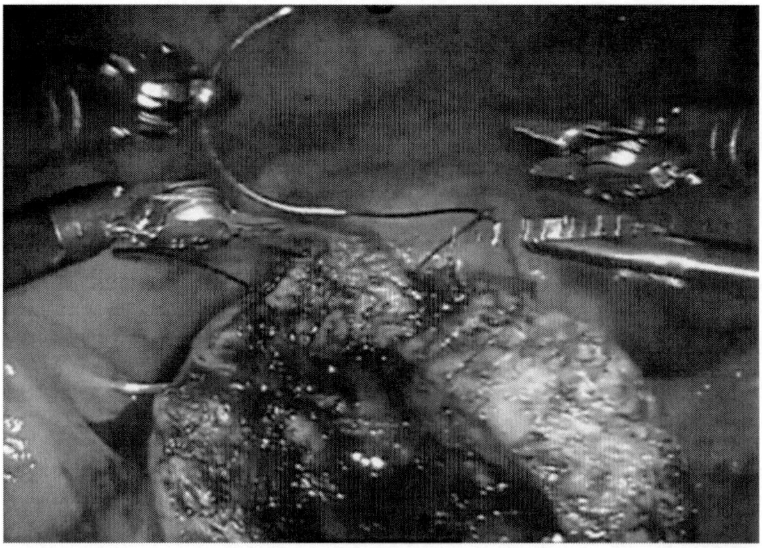

Hysterotomy closure.

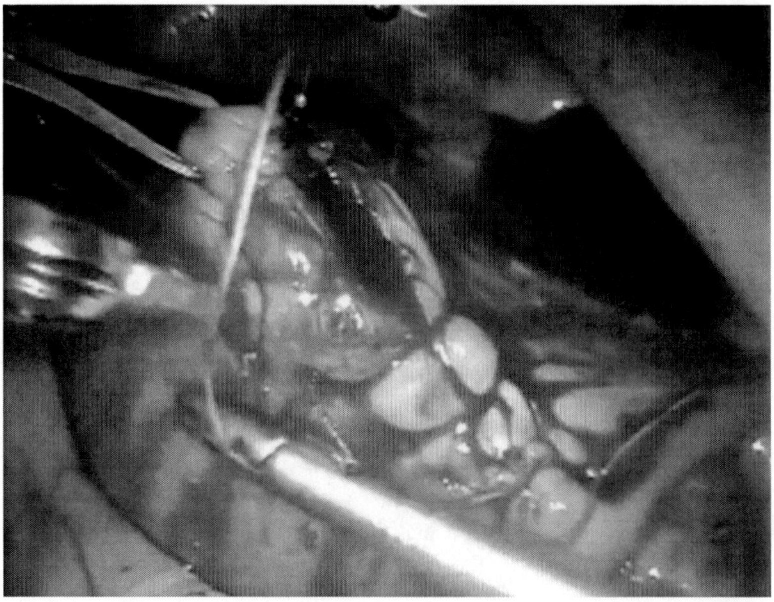

Hysterotomy closure.

- adhesion barrier onto the closed hysterotomy could be used to prevent future scar tissue formation
- specimen's morcellation and retrieval is achieved through assistant's port

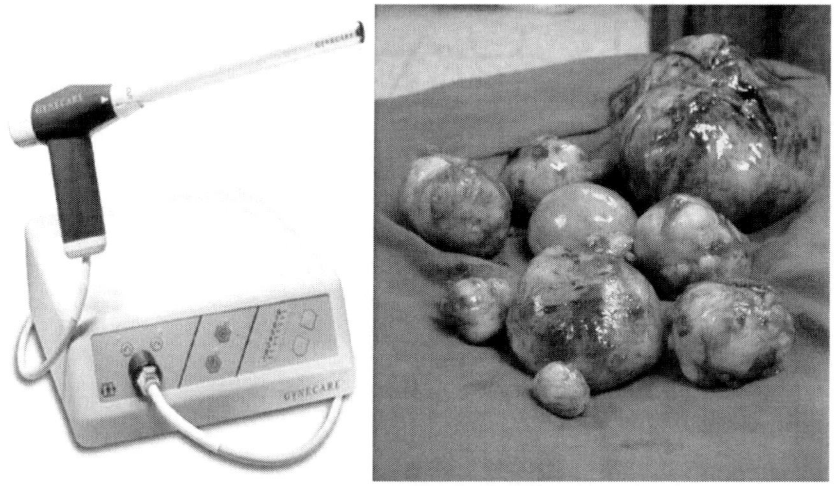

Morcellator and uterine fibroids.

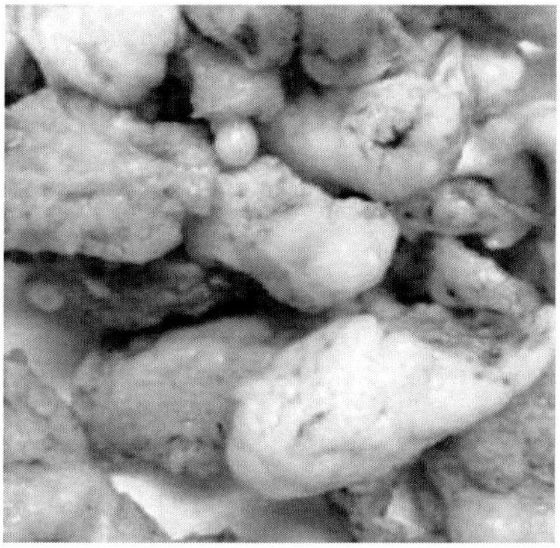

Specimen's morcellation.

Robotic Simple Hysterectomy

a) Blue dye injected on hours 12, 3, 6, 9 of the cervical to vaginal fornix edge
b) 2 vicryl sutures placed on the cervix.
c) Uterus instrumented with manipulator but balloon not inflated and cervical cap tied with the sutures.
d) Indwelling foley at outset.
e) Veress, pneumo and trocars.
f) Side docking. Uncomplicated instrumentation.
g) BIPOLAR diathermy at 40. Scissors in right main port with monopolar diathermy at 40 cut and coag. Cadiere or Maryland in 3rd arm.
h) Broads entered after incising with monopolar.
i) Ureters identified on both sides.
j) IP pedicles taken with bipolar and monopolar.

k) Rounds taken with bipolar and monopolar. UV fold peritoneum opened with monopolar.
l) Reflection of bladder.
m) Uterine vessels skeletalised and then taken with bipolar and monopolar.
n) Vagina entered anteriorly on top of the manipulator's cervical cap and dissection continued circumferentially using monopolar.
o) Uterine specimen extracted through vagina.
p) Glove with swab inserted in vagina to maintain pneumo.
q) Vaginal vault closed with continuous v-lock from right to left. No knot at the end.
r) Pelvis washed out.
s) Haemostasis confirmed.
t) Undocking.

Postoperative Care

- early mobilization and even same-day discharge are suggested.
- possible need for caesarean delivery in future pregnancies

Advantages of Robotic Approach

- three-dimensional (3D) view
- wrist-like motion of the robotic arms lower blood loss (even < 50 ml)
- fewer wound complications
- fewer urinary tract injuries
- minimal rates of conversion to open
- ideal for obese patients
- reduced length of hospital stay (around 24 hours)
- faster return to normal activities

Disadvantages:

- Cost
- Learning curve (operative time continues to decrease with increased experience)

Prognosis:

- 1/1000 fibroids can evolve in malignant lesion, particularly in leiomyosarcoma
- Patients who are not candidate for surgical treatment should be followed up both with clinical examination and ultrasonography

Chapter 13

Endometriosis

Definition:

- A benign process characterized by the presence and proliferation of endometrial tissue in sites outside the uterine cavity.

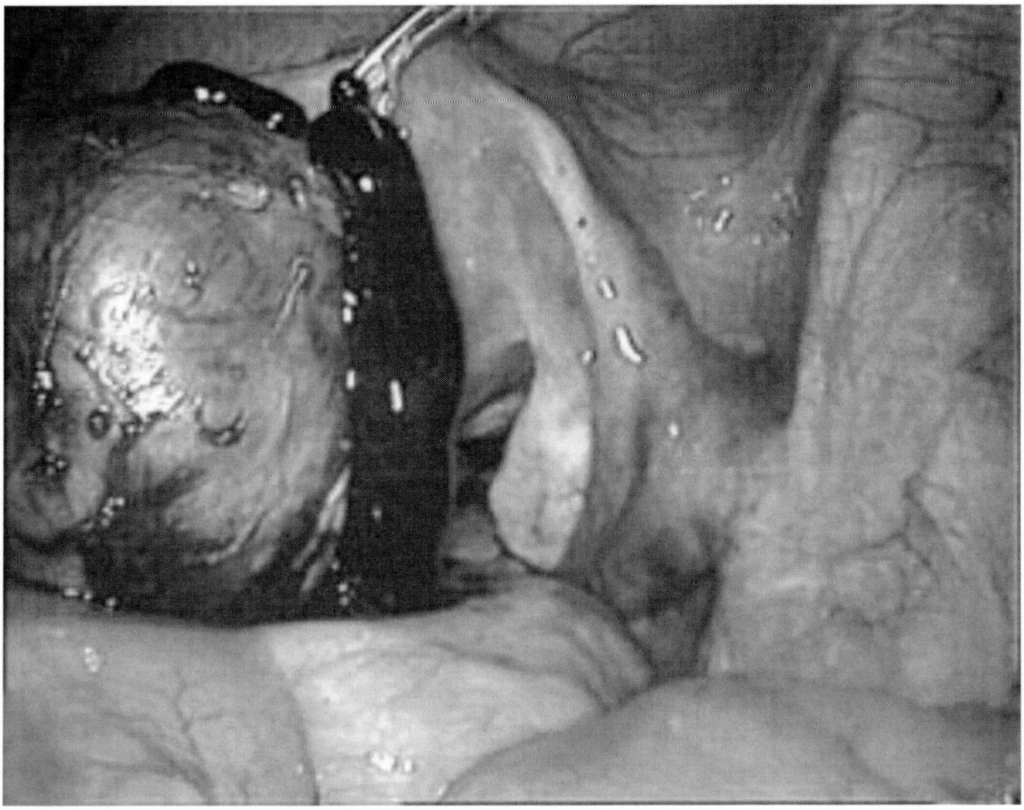

Endometrioma.

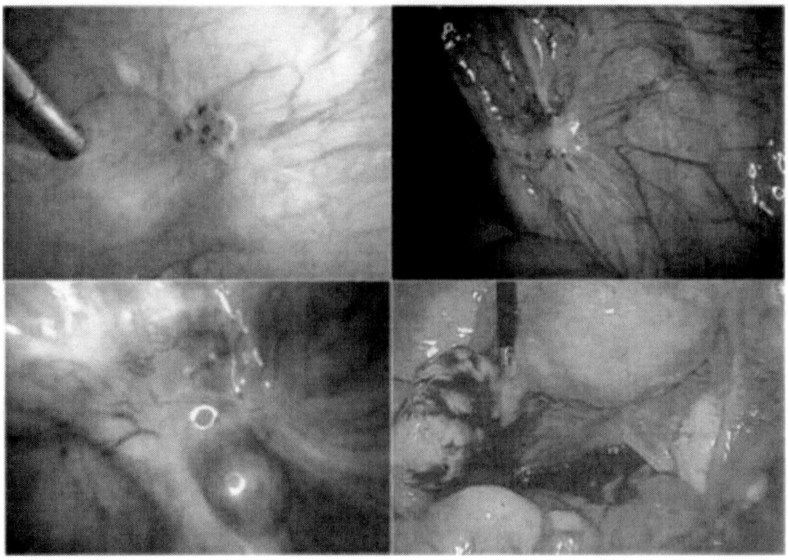

Endometriosis.

Incidence:

- <10% of premenopausal Caucasian women.
- 30% of women presenting with infertility.

Symptoms:

- asymptomatic
- cyclical pain
- dyspareunia
- secondary dysmenorrhea
- haematuria (in case of bladder involvement)
- rectal bleeding (in case of bowel involvement)

Diagnosis:

- through laparoscopy / laparotomy
- sigmoidoscopy / cystoscopy (in case of bowel / blabber involvement)

Staging (by American Society of Reproductive Medicine):

Stage	
I (minimal)	only superficial lesions and possibly a few filmy adhesions
II (mild)	deep lesions are present in the cul-de-sac
III (moderate)	presence of endometriomas on the ovary, more adhesions
IV (severe)	presence of large endometriomas, extensive adhesions

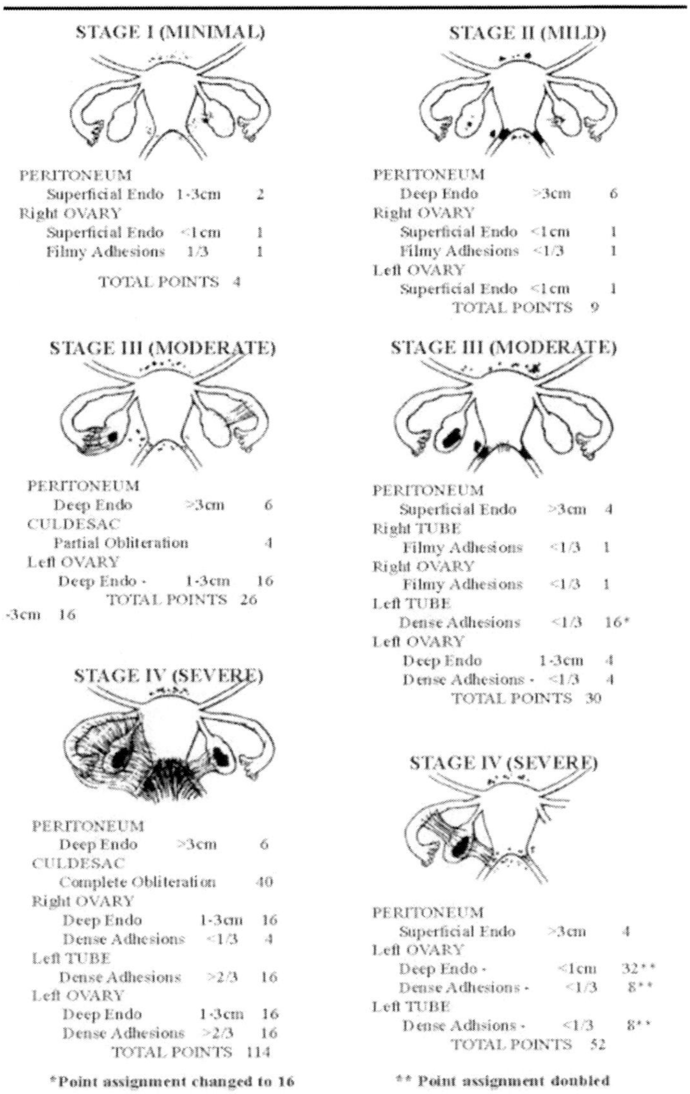

Staging of endometriosis.

Medical management:

- symptomatology improves in pregnancy
- oral contraceptive therapy (without intervals for withdrawal bleeds) mimics pregnancy
- progesterons, gestrinone, danazol and GnRH analogues suppress ovulation, relieving the symptoms

Surgical management:

- surgical treatment is advised when medical management is not successful or when there are present medical conditions which inhibit the use of hormone therapy

Surgical steps for robotic management:

a) bladder catheter placed to empty the bladder and control the urine output
b) cystoscopy plus/minus insertion of ureteral stents bilaterally if necessary
c) uterine manipulator to manipulate the uterus
d) exploration of the entire abdominal cavity to evaluate the extension of endometriotic lesions

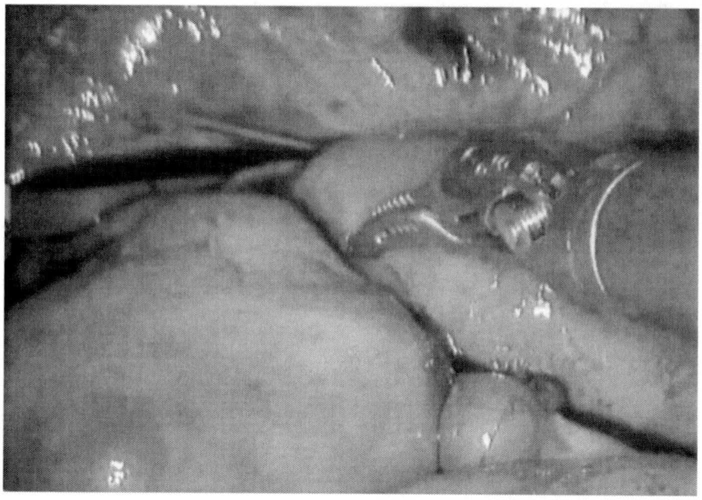

Exploration of the endometriotic lesions.

e) the robotic instruments used: monopolar scissors, bipolar forceps, a monopolar hook and one large needle holder
f) nerve-sparing approach
g) mobilisation of the ureters down to the level of the bladder
h) dissection starts, if necessary, with a complete, bilateral, salpingo-oophorectomy and the eventual excision of endometrioma(s)

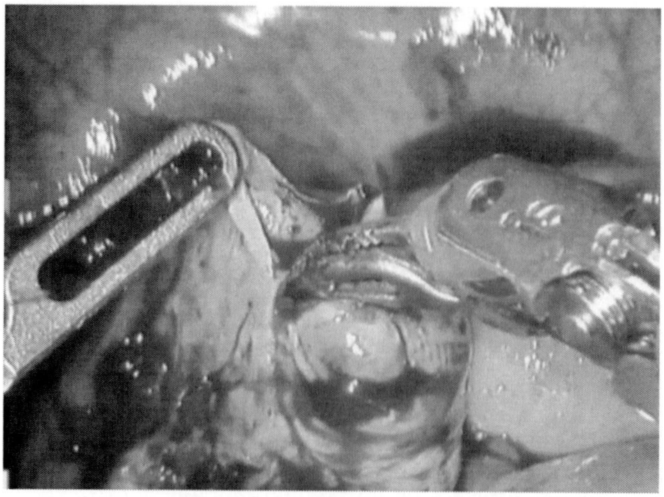

Excision of endometrioma.

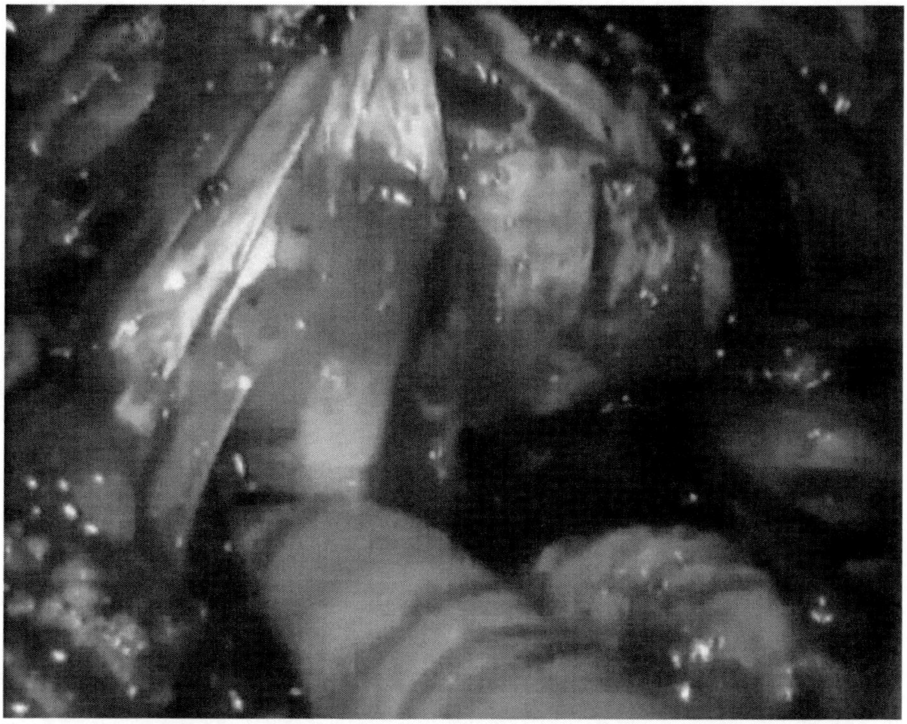

Excision of endometrioma.

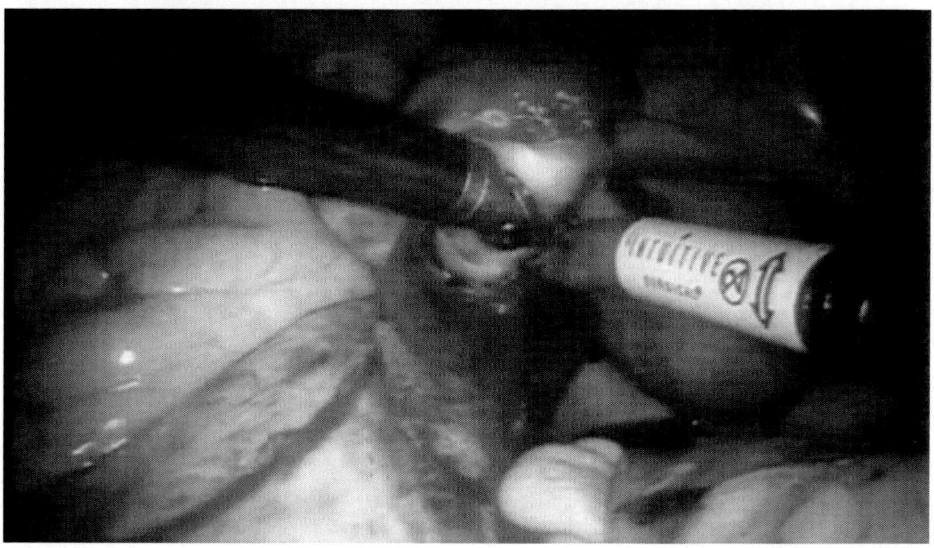

Excision of endometrioma.

i. excision of endometriotic nodules with or without stripping

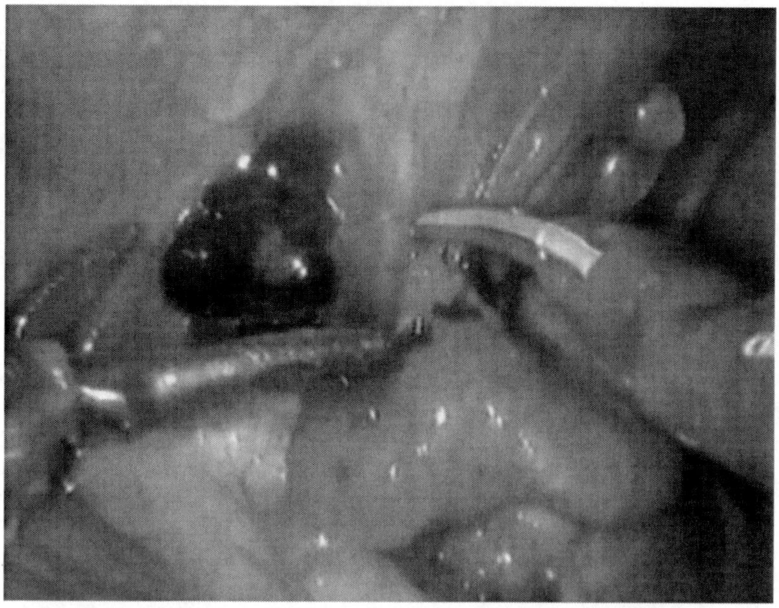

Excision of endometriotic nodules.

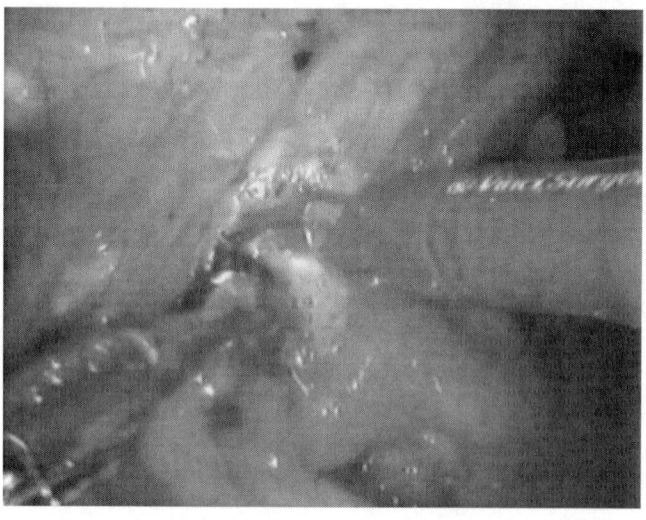

Excision of endometriotic nodules.

j. mobilisation of the sigmoid colon and opening of the retroperitoneum to identify the presacral fascia, the ureters, the uterine arteries and the hypogastric nerves
k. in case of a planned intestinal resection, extensive mobilization of the descending colon to identify the superior rectal artery
l. ureters and nerves are separated by the peritoneum and the Okabayashy pararectal space is developed up to the uterosacral ligaments or the puborectal portion of the levator ani muscle according to the position and caudal extension of the nodules
m. complete ureterolysis and parametrial resection in case of a lateral extension of the endometriotic nodule with involvement of periureteral/parametrial tissue

n. if an intestinal resection is not planned, separation of the nodule from the intestinal wall by the 'shaving technique'
o. reconstruction of the muscular portion of the rectal wall in cases involving rectal shaving by using 3/0, interrupted, absorbable monofilament sutures placed in the transverse direction to avoid narrowing the lumen
p. if necessary bowel segmental resection with an end-to-end anastomosis by using a rectally introduced circular stapler
q. ensure that there is no tension at the level of the anastomosis
r. integrity of the anastomosis tested by filling the rectum with blue solution and by an air test in a water-filled pelvis

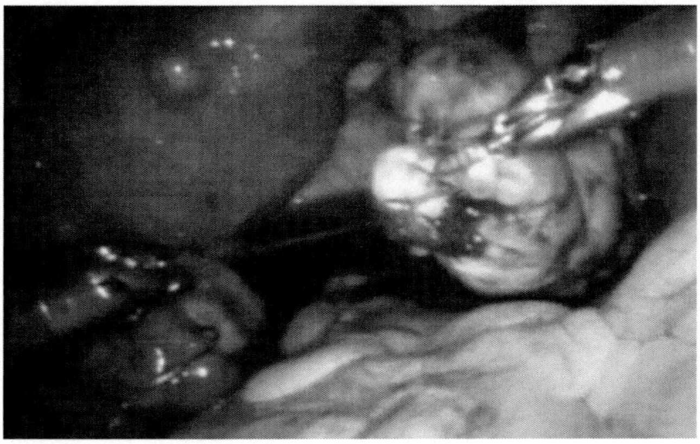

Excision of endometrioma.

Advantages of robotic approach:

- three-dimensional (3D) view
- wrist-like motion of the robotic arms lower blood loss (even < 50 ml)
- fewer wound complications
- fewer urinary tract injuries
- minimal rates of conversion to open
- ideal for obese patients
- reduced length of hospital stay (around 24 hours)
- faster return to normal activities

Disadvantages:

- Cost
- Learning curve (operative time continues to decrease with increased experience)

Prognosis:

- Endometriosis recurrence occurs at a rate of 20 to 40% within 5 years period after conservative surgery.
- Follow up of patients consists of clinical examinations and ultrasonography.
- Childbirth decreases recurrence of endometriosis. Vaginal birth has lower endometriosis recurrence rates in comparison with caesarean section

Chapter 14

Robotic Management of Ectopic Pregnancy

a. Salpingectomy (if the tube has already ruptured as a result of an ectopic pregnancy)

- Progressively coagulating and cutting the mesosalpinx, starting from the fimbriated end and advancing toward the proximal isthmic portion of the tube
- Tube separated from the uterus

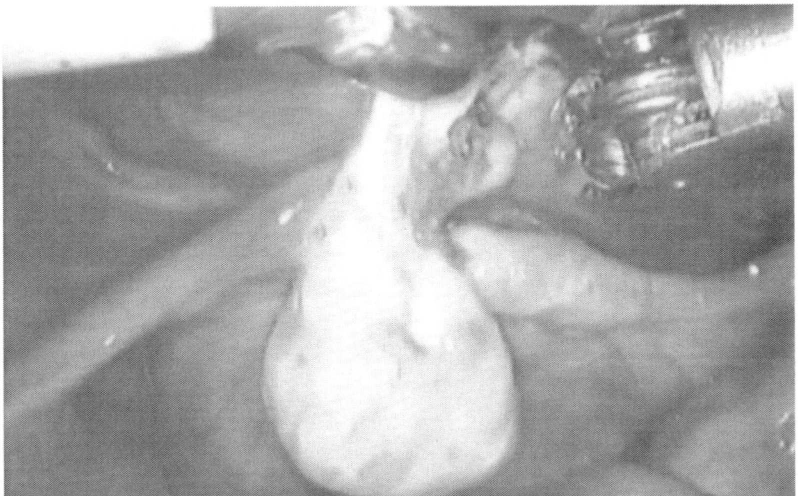

Salpingectomy.

Indications:

- Ruptured ectopic pregnancy
- Future fertility not desired - sterilization.
- Ectopic pregnancy as a result of failure of sterilization.
- Previous tubal reconstruction

- Uncontrollable bleeding after salpingotomy.
- Ectopic pregnancy in the blind-ending distal segment after a previous partial salpingectomy.
- Chronic tubal pregnancy.

b. Salpingotomy

Usually ectopic pregnancies in the ampulla are usually located between the lumen and the serosa

- Vasopressin(10 or 20 IU in 50 mL of normal saline) is injected into the fallopian tube to minimize the amount of bleeding
- Avoid intravascular injection
- Linear incision of the ante-mesosalpingeal wall of the tube with monopolar curved scissors
- Removal of conception products
- Any bleeding sites can be treated by suturing or by applying pressure with forceps
- The incision is not sutured (closure by secondary intent)

Chapter 15

Robotic Tubal Anastomosis

Indication: Patients with history of tubal sterilization with a desire for more children (need for reversal)

Setup:

Modified-lithotomy position using Allen stirrups with the arms tucked to each side.

Padding is used to protect both arms and legs.

To avoid sliding, an antiskid bean bag secured to the operating table could be used.

Trendelenburg position is asked until the small bowel and sigmoid are displaced out of the pelvis before docking.

Uterine manipulator with a side channel for injection of indigo carmine could be used.

Side Docking

Ports positioning: 12-mm umbilical port for the camera and two 8-mm side ports lateral and at 15 degrees below the umbilical one, placed in the midaxillary line. A 5-mm to 10-mm accessory fourth port placed on the left side between the umbilicus and the anterior superior iliac spine used for suction irrigation and introduction or removal of sutures and needles. For tubal anastomosis, the assistant's trocar should be placed lower to allow direct visualization for the introduction of the very small needles used in order to avoid losing them. Third robotic arm trocar could be used especially in obese patients or cases with a lot of adhesions.

Robotic instruments that could be used are: An EndoWrist PK grasper, an EndoWristmonopolar hook, EndoWristmonopolar scissors, Endo-WristPrograsper, EndoWrist needle holder.

No cautery is used on the muscularis-mucosal layer

Surgical Technique

c) subserosal injection of vasopressin diluted 20U in 200mL of normal saline in both proximal and distal ends and in the mesosalpinx to facilitate subsequent dissection of both ends and hemostasis

d) injection of indigo carmine dye transcervically for identification of the proximal tubal portion and exclusion of proximal tubal obstruction
e) a probe is placed through the fimbriated end of the distal portion and indigo carmine injected to identify the distal anastomosis site
f) the serosal covering of the proximal and distal anastomosis site is incised with monopolar cautery
g) microscissors can be used to cut the muscularis-mucosal portion of the tube to open the proximal and distal ends of the tube
h) mesosalpinx is approximated using a series of 6-0 Vicryl stitches to bridge the gap between the 2 ends of the fallopian tube and to facilitate subsequent suturing in a way to prevent tension on the anastomosis site
i) if there is a major discrepancy in size between the proximal and distal anastomosis site, a stent is placed to facilitate the suturing of the two ends

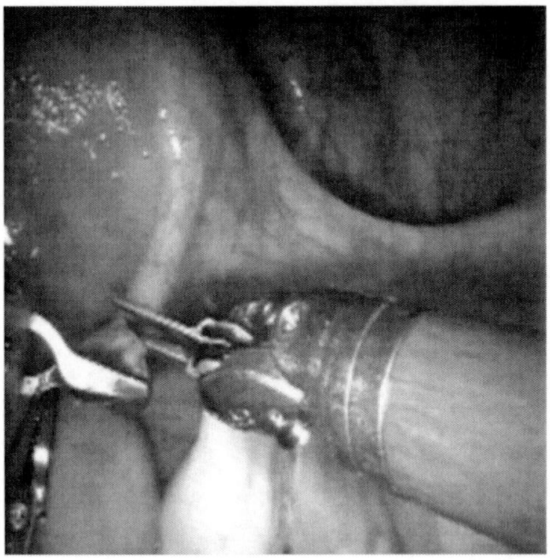

Steps of tubal anastomosis.

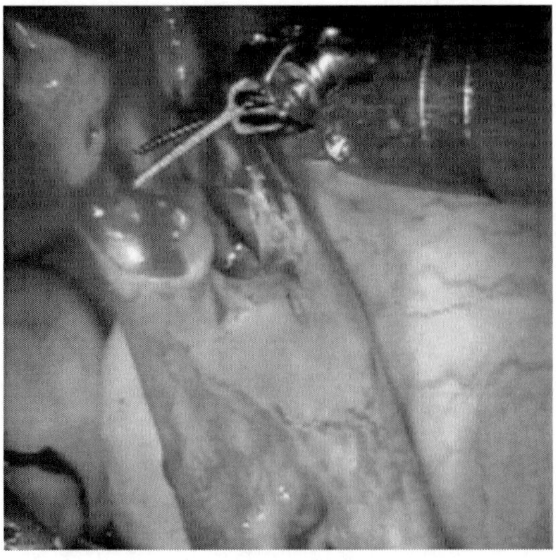

Steps of tubal anastomosis.

k) the mucosal and muscular layers of the tubal segments are sutured with 4 interrupted 8-0 Vicryl sutures by moving both hands gently and simultaneously while tying the knot to avoid damaging the needle or suture (first suture at 6 o'clock with the knot outside of the lumen, and tied with the intracorporeal knot tying technique, second, third and fourth sutures at 3, 9 and 12 o'clock, respectively)

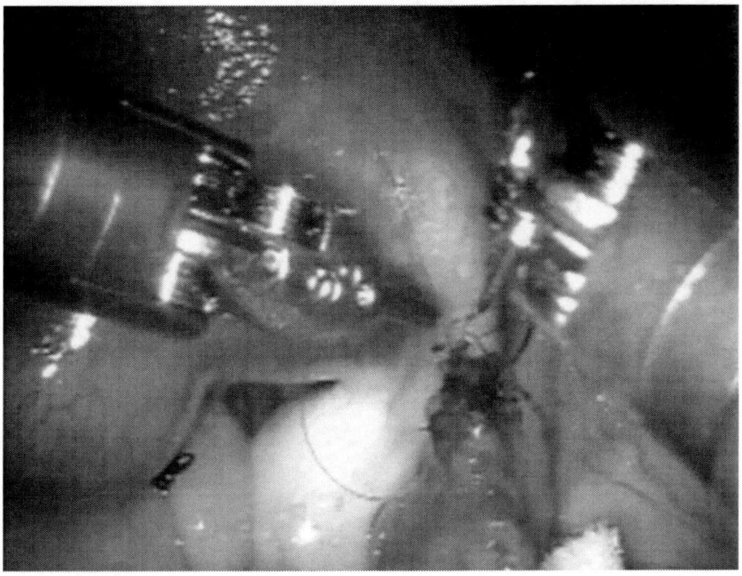

Steps of tubal anastomosis.

l) attention is necessary to avoid misalignment or rotation of the distal tubal segment along its longitudinal axis

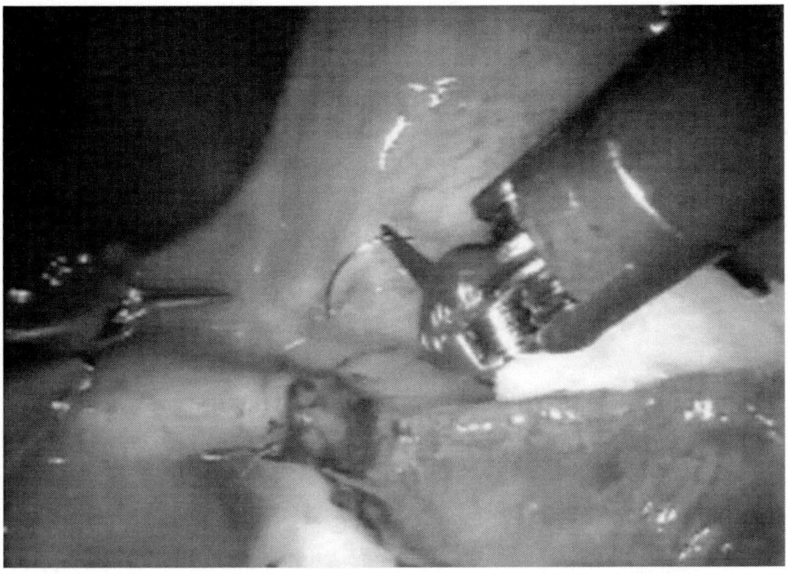

Steps of tubal anastomosis.

m) serosa is closed separately with 7-0 Vicryl sutures

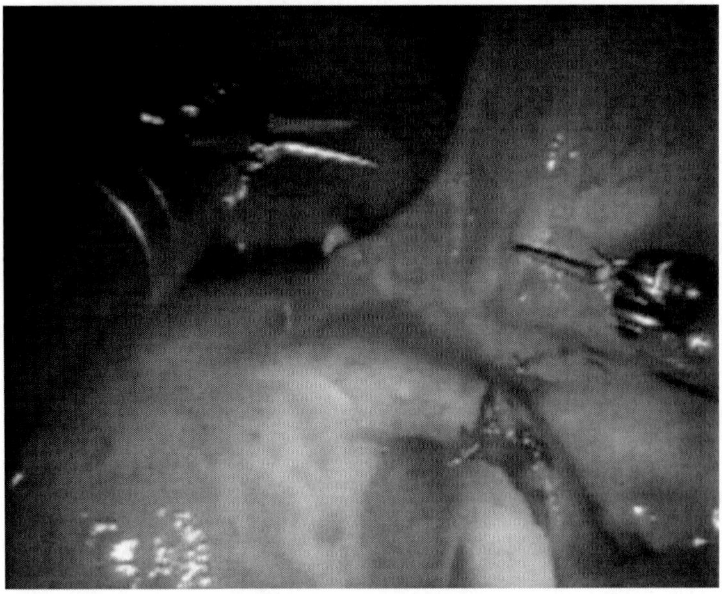

Steps of tubal anastomosis.

n) success of the procedure is checked with chromotubation

Postoperative Course

Foley catheter removed at the end of the procedure.

Oral intake, including oral medications on the same day of the operation, and patients are allowed to ambulate as soon as possible.

Postoperative visit at 6 weeks.

Chapter 16

Sacrocolpopexy

- sacrocolpopexy or sacral colpopexy is defined as the surgical technique utilized for the repair of pelvic organ prolapse.
- In post-menopausal women, the prevalence of pelvic organ prolapse ranges between 31 to 41.1% while the risk for a woman during her life to undergo an operation for pelvic organ prolapse is 11 to 19%.
- The most important risk factors for pelvic organ prolapse include:

a) Age
b) Race (Hispanic)
c) Body mass index
d) Parity
e) Gravidity
f) The number of vaginal deliveries
g) Chronic obstructive pulmonary disease
h) Delivery of macrosomic infants
i) Constipation
j) Daily strenuous activity

Surgical Steps of Robotic Sacrocolpopexy

- The patient is placed in low lithotomy position in stirrups. The patient is secured to the table in steep Trendelenburg position.
- Intravenous prophylactic antibiotic
- Foley catheter
- Five trocar sites are used: A 12-mm trocar is placed at the level of the umbilicus for the camera. Another10-mm trocar is placed on the right side, approximately 6 to 8 cm lateral to the umbilical port.
- A 5-mm trocar is placed on the left side, contralateral at the 10-mm port. A supplementary 5-mm port is positioned on the right side about 5 cm superior and medially to the anterior superior iliac spine. The final fifth assistant trocar can be

positioned on the left side about 5 cm superior and medially to the anterior superior iliac spine. The assistant of the surgeon stands on the patient's left.

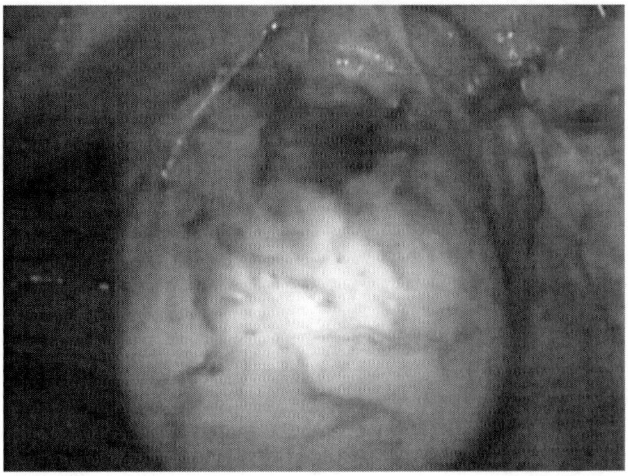

Bladder resection.

- A manipulator is used vaginally.
- Pneumoperitoneum
- Packing away the bowel from the field.

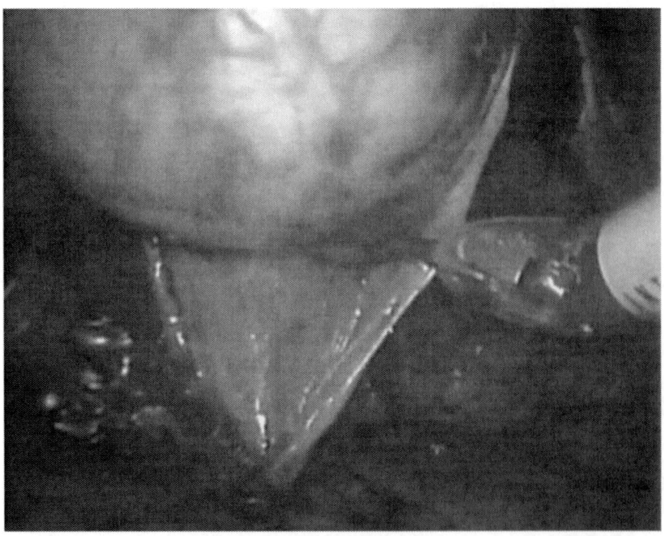

Bladder resection.

- Dissection of the bladder away from the anterior vagina along the vesicovaginal septum; continued posteriorly to separate the vagina from the rectum along the rectovaginal septum
- Exposure of retroperitoneal space

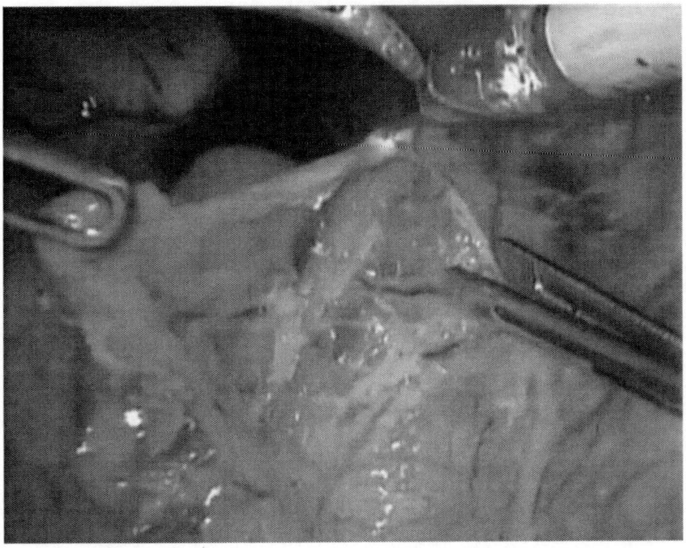

Exposure of retroperitoneal space.

- Identification of the point for fixation of the mesh on the sacral promontory.
- A Y-shaped mesh is utilized to sustain the vaginal wall and to suspend the anterior and posterior vaginal wall to the sacral promontory.

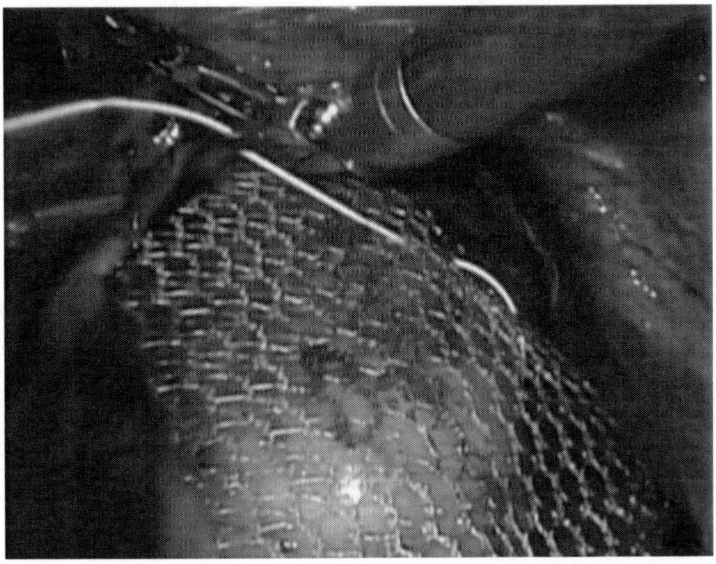

Mesh fixation.

- The mesh can be fixed, in a tension-free manner, with the use of 2-0 non absorbable monofilament sutures. Otherwise, bone anchoring devices can be used to fix the mesh to the sacral promontory.

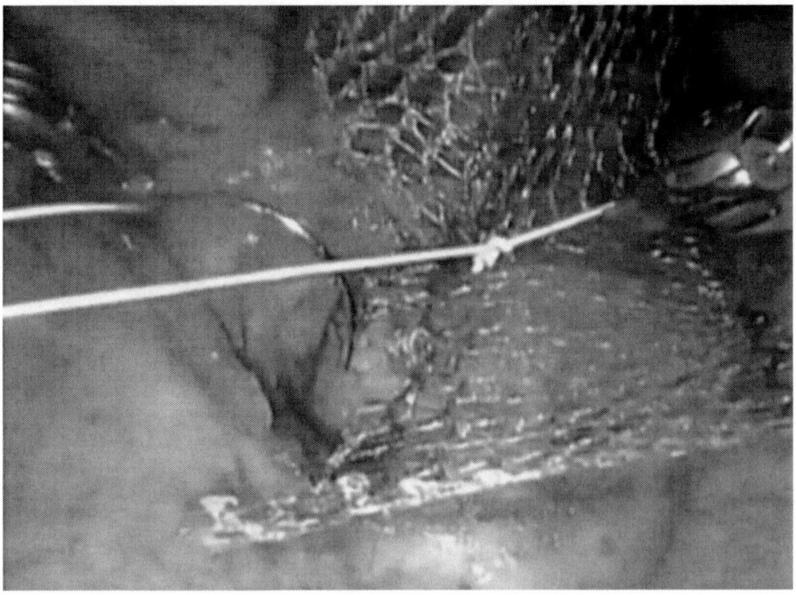

Mesh fixation.

- Peritoneal closure over the mesh.

Chapter 17

Endometrial Cancer: Robotic Simple Hysterectomy

Incidence:

- the most common gynaecological malignancy
- median age: 63 years

Risk factors:

- early onset of menstruation
- obesity
- nulliparity
- late menopause
- diabetes mellitus
- hypertension
- infertility
- unopposed estrogen exposure
- tamoxifen
- Lynch syndrome type II

Presenting symptom: abnormal uterine bleeding in 90% of the cases

Diagnosis:

- U/S: endometrial thickness, using a cut-off point of 3 or 4 mm
- endometrial sampling (Pipelle, Uterobrush, dilatation and curettage (D&C) – hysteroscopy)

Preoperative evaluation:

- clinical and gynecological examination

- transvaginal ultrasound
- FBC, U&E, LFT
- CT abdomen-pelvis
- MRI abdomen-pelvis
- PET/CT

Histology: Two main types: Type I or endometrioid adenocarcinomas represent 80% of endometrial cancers. Type II or non endometrioid endometrial cancers

FIGO staging 2009:

Stage	
I	Tumor confined to the corpus uteri
Ia	No or less than half myometrial invasion
Ib	Invasion equal to or more than half of the myometrium
II	Tumor invades cervical stroma, but does not extend beyond the uterus
III	Local and/or regional spread of the tumor
IIIa	Tumor invades the serosa of the corpus uteri and/or adnexae
IIIb	Vaginal and/or parametrial involvement
IIIc	Metastasis to pelvic and/or para-aortic lymph nodes
	III C1 Positive pelvic nodes
	III C2 Positive para-aortic lymph nodes with or without positive pelvic lymph nodes
IV	Tumor invades bladder and/or bowel mucosa, and/or distant metastases
IVa	Tumor invasion of bladder and/or bowel mucosa
IVb	Distant metastases, including intra-abdominal metastases and/or inguinal lymph nodes

Surgical management:

1. standard approach for stage I endometrial cancer: total hysterectomy, bilateral salpingo-oophorectomy, washings with or without lymphadenectomy. Systematic pelvic lymphadenectomy is an issue of current debate. Lymphadenectomy is highly important in determining a patient's prognosis and in tailoring adjuvant treatment. Para-aortic lymphadenectomy is also considered in stage II.
2. Papillary serous and clear cell cancers require complete staging (total hysterectomy, bilateral salpingo-oophorectomy, pelvic and para-aortic lymphadenectomy, omentectomy, appendicectomy and peritoneal biopsies).

Choice of Incision:

- Traditionally, abdominally, using an open technique, via a low transverse or vertical midline incision

- laparoscopic hysterectomy and bilateral salpingo-oophorectomy
- robotic hysterectomy and bilateral salpingo-oophorectomy

Surgical steps for robotic simple hysterectomy:

a) 2 vicryl sutures on the cervix.
b) Uterus instrumented with manipulator but balloon not inflated and cervical cap tied with the sutures.
c) Indwelling foley at outset.
d) Veress, pneumo and trocars.
e) Side docking. Uncomplicated instrumentation.
f) Bipolar diathermy at 40. Scissors in right main port with monopolar diathermy at 40 cut and coag. Cadiere or Maryland in 3rd arm.
g) Broads entered after incising with monopolar.
h) Ureters identified on both sides.
i) IP pedicles taken with bipolar and monopolar.
j) Rounds taken with bipolar and monopolar. UV fold peritoneum with monopolar.
k) Reflection of bladder.
l) Uterine vessels skeletalised and then taken with bipolar and monopolar.
m) Vagina entered anteriorly on top of the manipulator's cervical cap and dissection continued circumferentially using monopolar.
n) Uterine specimen extracted through vagina.
o) Glove with swab inserted in vagina to maintain pneumo.
p) Vaginal vault closed with continuous v-lock from right to left. No knot at the end.
q) Pelvis washed out.
r) Haemostasis confirmed.
s) Undocking.

Surgical steps for robotic pelvic lymph node sampling:

a) Ureters identified on both sides.
b) Pelvic side wall entered overlying the external iliac vessels.
c) Uncomplicated and thorough dissection of lymph nodes from the external iliac vessels up to the bifurcation of the common iliac vessels.
d) Boundaries of pelvic lymph node dissection:

    - Lateral: genitofemoral nerve
    - Medial: ureter
    - Inferior: deep iliac circumflex vein

Superior: inferior mesenteric artery

a) Pelvic lymph nodes extracted through the port in laparoscopic bags.

Step-by-step robotic hysterectomy and bilateral salpingo-oophorectomy

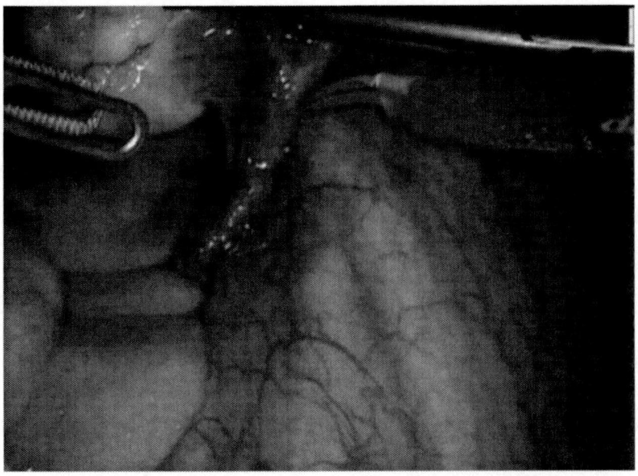

Ureters identified on both sides.

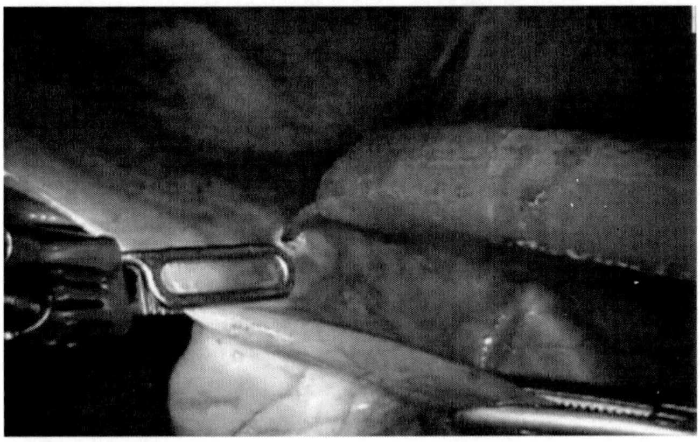

Broads entered after incising with monopolar.

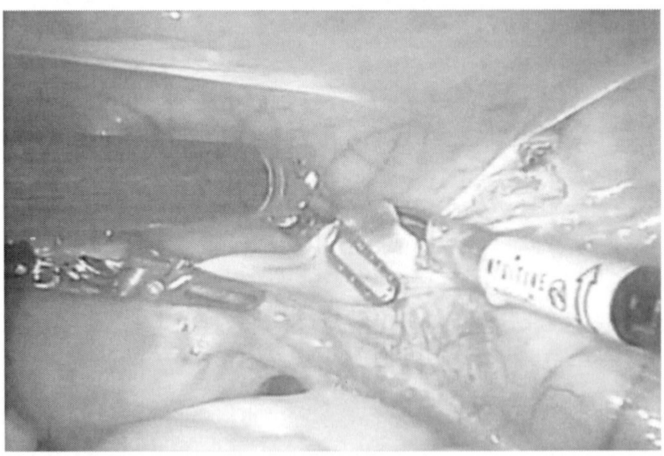

Rounds taken with bipolar and monopolar. UV fold peritoneum with monopolar.

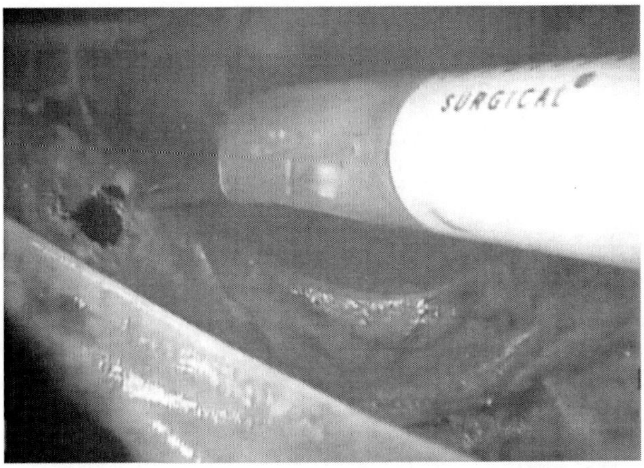

IP pedicles taken with bipolar and monopolar.

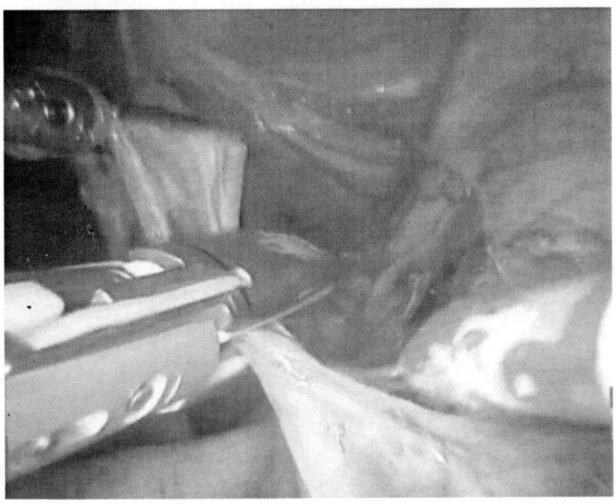

IP pedicles taken with bipolar and monopolar.

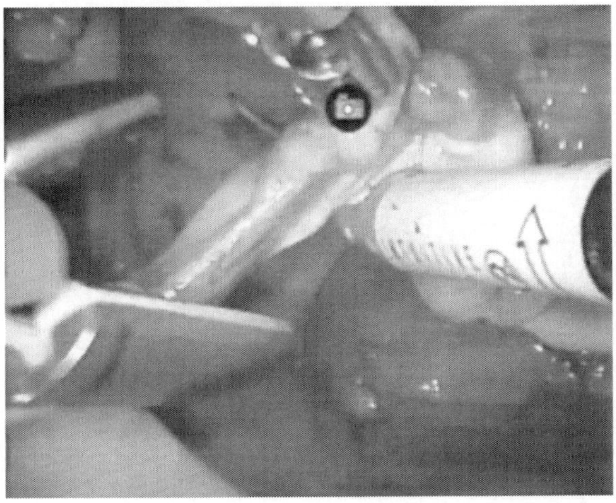

IP pedicles taken with bipolar and monopolar.

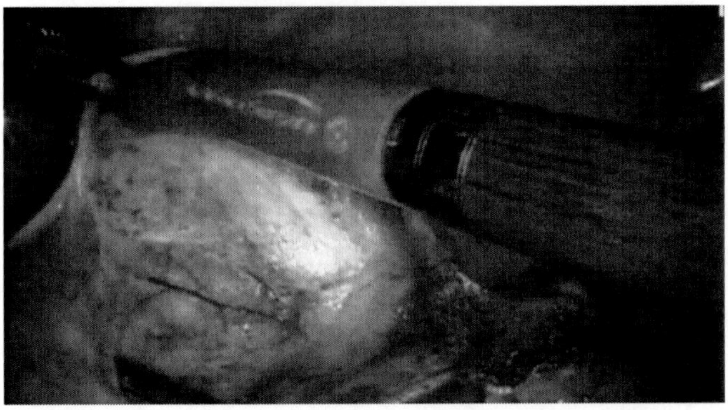

Reflection of bladder.

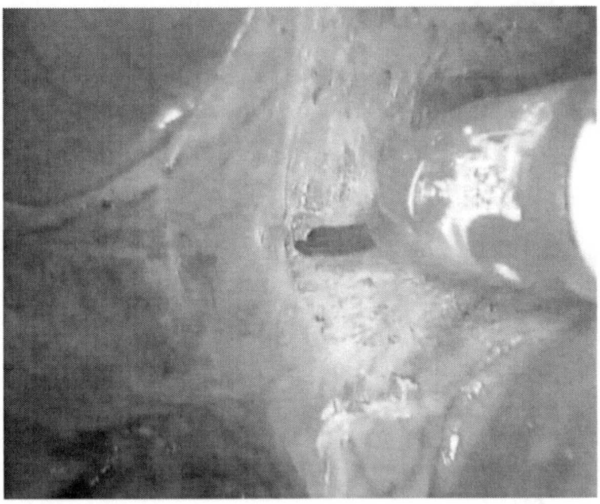

Reflection of bladder.

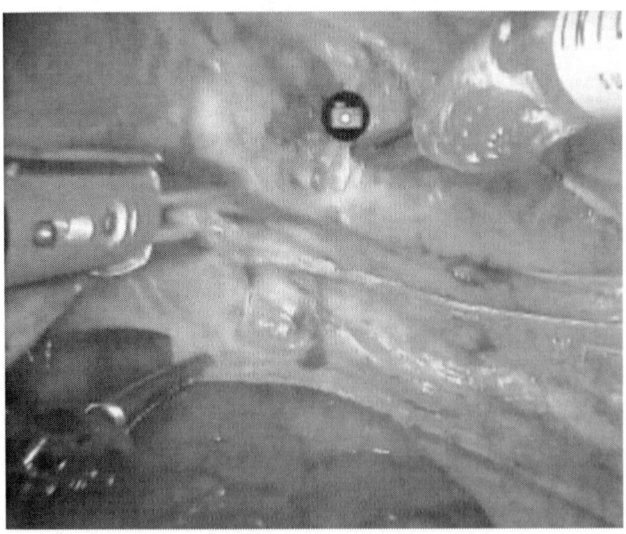

Uterine vessels skeletalised and then taken with bipolar and monopolar.

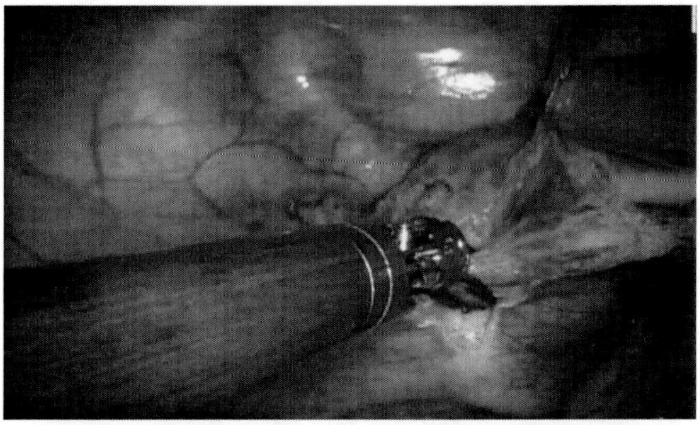

Uterine vessels skeletalised and then taken with bipolar and monopolar.

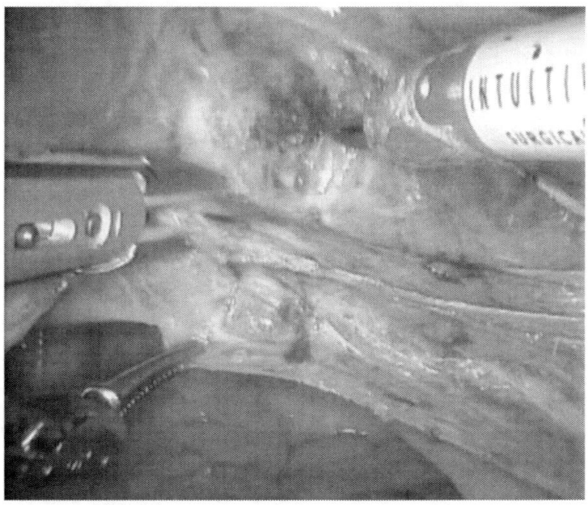

Uterine vessels skeletalised and then taken with bipolar and monopolar.

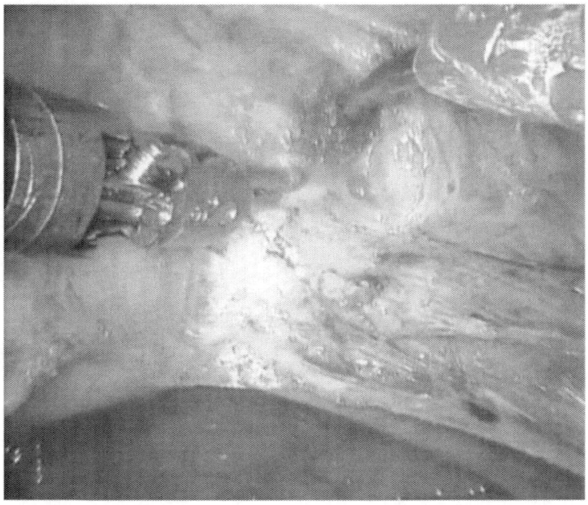

Uterine vessels skeletalised and then taken with bipolar and monopolar.

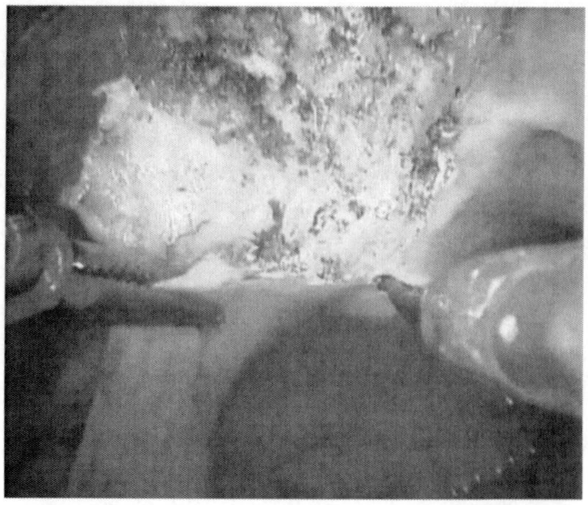

Uterine vessels skeletalised and then taken with bipolar and monopolar.

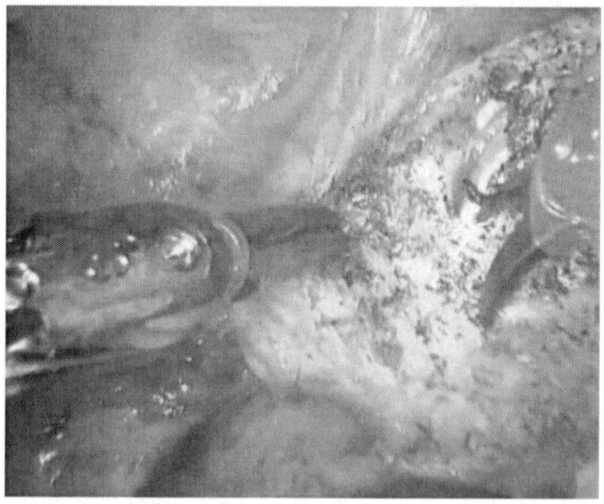

Vagina entered anteriorly on top of the manipulator's cervical cap and dissection continued circumferentially using monopolar.

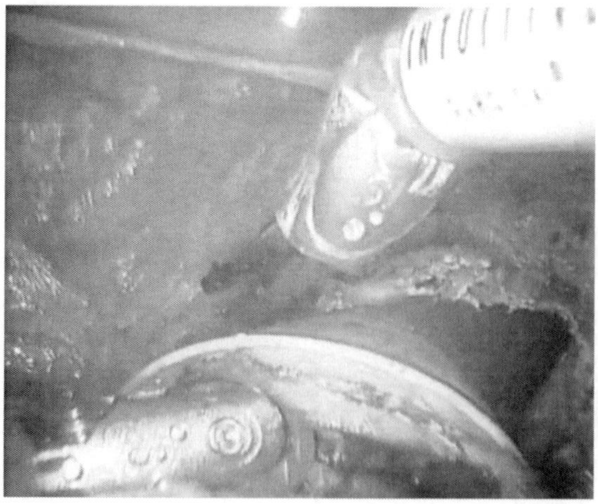

Vagina entered anteriorly on top of the manipulator's cervical cap and dissection continued circumferentially using monopolar.

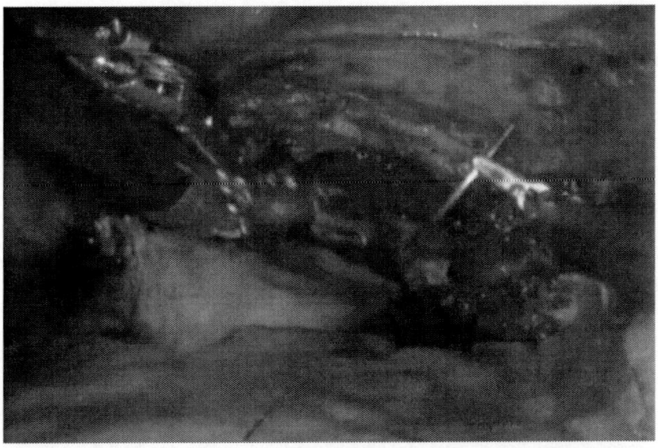

Vaginal vault closed with continuous v-lock from right to left. No knot at the end.

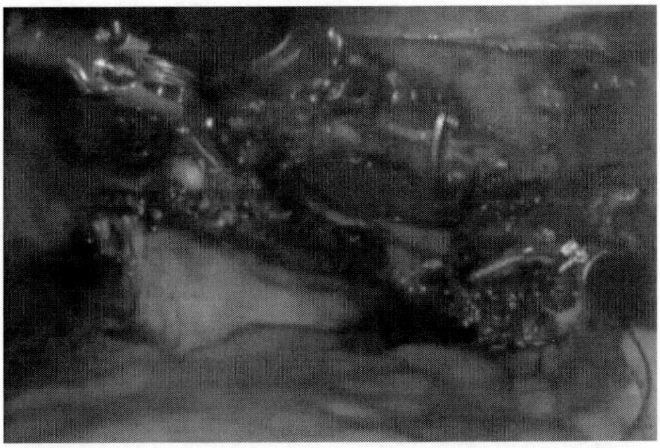

Vaginal vault closed with continuous v-lock from right to left. No knot at the end.

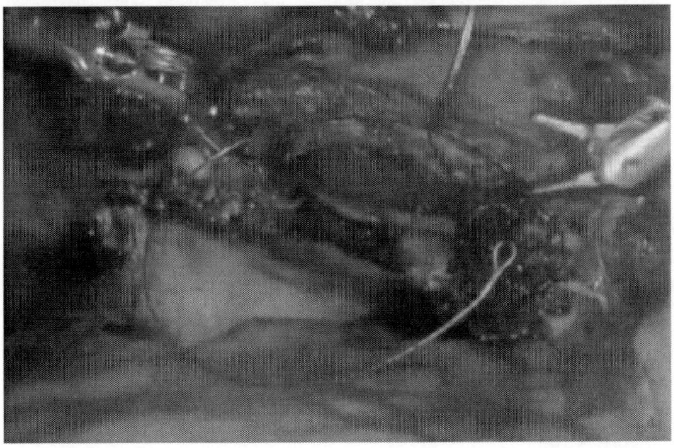

Vaginal vault closed with continuous v-lock from right to left. No knot at the end.

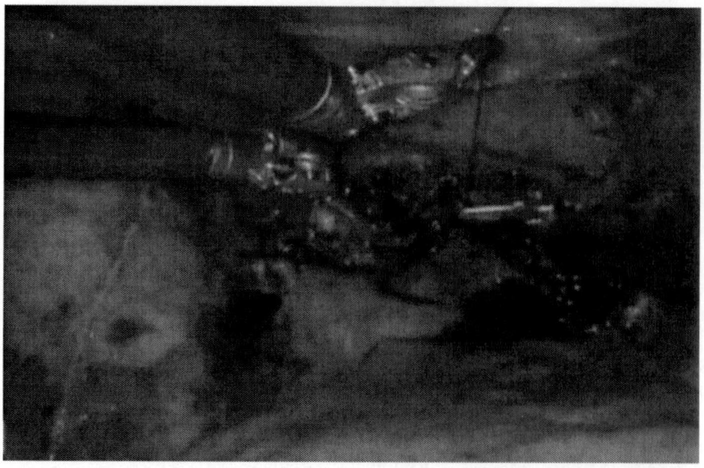

Vaginal vault closed with continuous v-lock from right to left. No knot at the end.

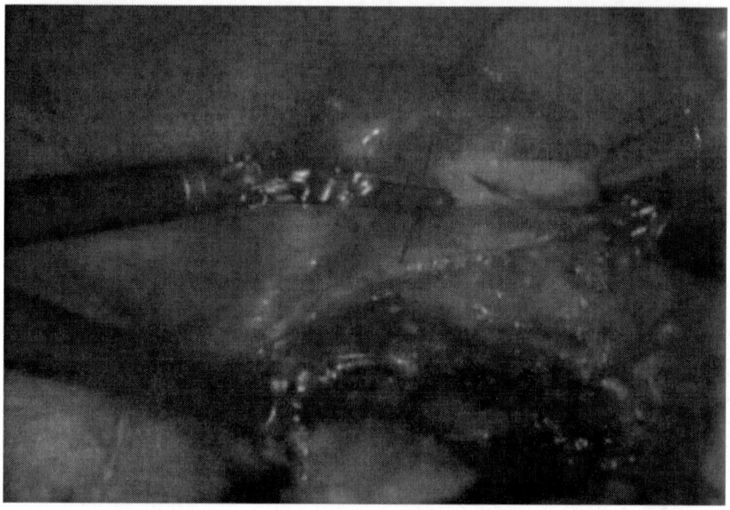

Vaginal vault closed with continuous v-lock from right to left. No knot at the end.

Advantages of robotic approach:

- three-dimensional (3D) view
- wrist-like motion of the robotic arms lower blood loss (even < 50 ml)
- higher lymph node retrieval
- fewer wound complications
- fewer urinary tract injuries
- minimal rates of conversion to open
- ideal for obese patients
- reduced length of hospital stay (from 1 to 1.6 days)
- faster return to normal activities

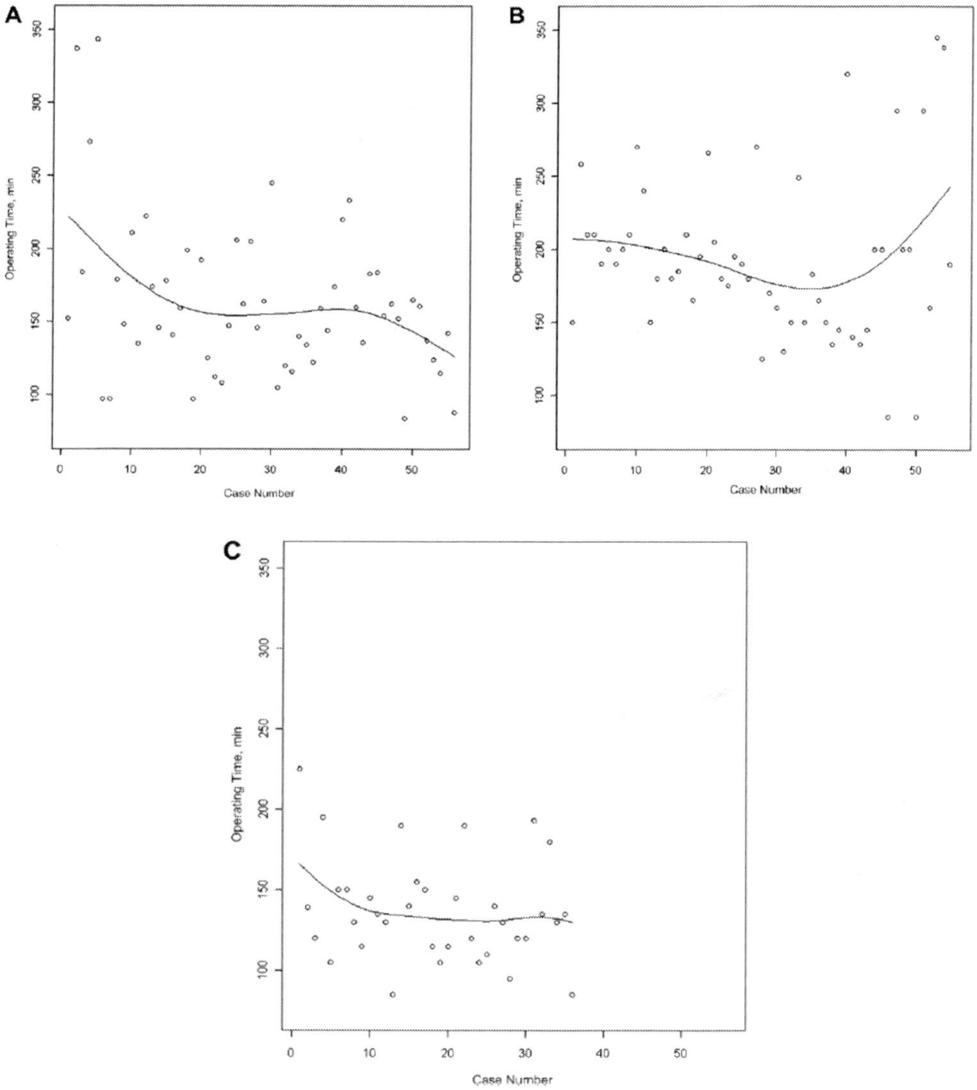

Reference: Lim PC et al Learning curve and surgical outcome for robotic-assisted hysterectomy with lymphadenectomy: case-matched controlled comparison with laparoscopy and laparotomy for treatment of endometrial cancer. J Minim Invas Gynecol 2010;17(6): 739-748.

Number of patients: Robotic hysterectomy (A): 56. Laparoscopic hysterectomy (B): 56, Open hysterectomy (C): 38.

Disadvantages:

- Cost
- Learning curve (operative time continues to decrease with increased experience)

Follow-up: every 3 months the first 2 years, then every 6 months until 5 years

Prognosis:

- overall 5-year survival rate in women with endometrial cancer is 83% (62% for clear cell and 53% for papillary carcinomas)
- affected by histological subtype, grade 3 histology, myometrial invasion ≥50%, LVSI, lymph node metastases and tumor diameter >2 cm

Chapter 18

Cervical Cancer: Robotic Radical Hysterectomy

Incidence:

- the second most common type of neoplasia among women between 15 to 44 years old
- cervical cancer can be managed with the combined use of surgery with or without radiotherapy/chemotherapy; the treatment strategy depends on the clinical stage of the cancer and whether there is recurrence

Aetiology:

- human papillomavirus (HPV) (types 16 / 18 and 31 / 45 are responsible for 75% and 10% of cervical cancer globally, respectively)
- smoking has been also associated with cervical cancer

Symptoms:

- asymptomatic (detected by screening programmes)
- vaginal bleeding (especially postcoital bleeding) or vaginal discharge

Diagnosis:

- Pap smear (Papanicolaou test) can be used as a screening test even though there are up to 50% false negative results.
- colposcopy
- conization and tissue biopsy

Preoperative evaluation:

- clinical and gynecological examination
- transvaginal ultrasound
- FBC, U&E, LFT
- CT abdomen-pelvis
- MRI abdomen-pelvis
- PET/CT

Histology:

- squamous cell tumors (90%)
- adenocarcinomas (10%)

FIGO staging:

Stage 0:	The carcinoma is confined to the surface layer of the cervix. Also called carcinoma in situ (CIS).
Stage I:	The carcinoma has grown deeper into the cervix, but has not spread beyond it (extension to the corpus would be disregarded).
Stage IA:	Invasive carcinoma which can be diagnosed only by microscopy, with deepest invasion <5 mm and the largest extension <7 mm.
Stage IA1:	Measured stromal invasion of <3.0 mm in depth and extension of <7.0 mm.
Stage IA2:	Measured stromal invasion of >3.0 mm and not >5.0 mm with an extension of not >7.0 mm.
Stage IB:	Clinically visible lesions limited to the cervix uteri or pre-clinical cancers greater than stage IA.
Stage IB1:	Clinically visible lesion <4.0 cm in greatest dimension.
Stage IB2:	Clinically visible lesion >4.0 cm in greatest dimension.
Stage II:	Cervical carcinoma invades beyond the uterus, but not to the pelvic wall or to the lower third of the vagina.
Stage IIA:	Without parametrial invasion.
Stage IIA1:	Clinically visible lesion <4.0 cm in greatest dimension.
Stage IIA2:	Clinically visible lesion >4.0 cm in greatest dimension.
Stage IIB:	With obvious parametrial invasion.
Stage III:	The tumour extends to the pelvic wall and/or involves lower third of the vagina and/or causes hydronephrosis or non-functioning kidney.
Stage IIIA:	Tumour involves lower third of the vagina, with no extension to the pelvic wall.
Stage IIIB:	Extension to the pelvic wall and/or hydronephrosis or non-functioning kidney.
Stage IV:	The carcinoma has extended beyond the true pelvis or has involved (biopsy proven) the mucosa of the bladder or rectum. A bullous oedema, as such, does not permit a case to be allotted to Stage IV.
Stage IVA:	Spread of the growth to adjacent organs.
Stage IVB:	Spread to distant organs.

Surgical management:

- In stage Ia1, conization is considered as curative.
- For disease stage Ib-IIa, radical hysterectomy is considered the treatment. Often two stage procedure is offered initially with bilateral pelvic lymphadenopathy to assess the possible nodal infiltration followed by radical hysterectomy.

Evolution of surgical treatment of cervical cancer

1652	Pares & Talipius	Cervical amputation
1801-1808	Osiander	Eight cervical amputation
1813	Langenbeck	Vaginal hysterectomy
1878	Freund	Abdominal hysterectomy
1895	Ries & Clark	Radical hysterectomy/ lymphadenectomy
1900	Wertheim	Radical abdominal hysterectomy
1902	Schauta	Radical vaginal hysterectomy
1943	Taussig	Surgical treatment& radiation
1944	Meigs	Radical hysterectomy / lymphadenectomy
1987	Dargent	Coelio-Schauta's radical vaginal hysterectomy extraperitoneal lymphadenectomy
1988	Sakamoto	Nerve sparing radical hysterectomy
1990	Canis	Laparoscopic radical hysterectomy
1991	Querleu	Coelio- Schauta's radical vaginal hysterectomy transperitoneal lymphadenectomy
1992	Nezhat	Laparoscopic radical hysterectomy
1994	Dargent	Radical vaginal trachelectomy
1997	Smith	Radical abdominal trachelectomy
1998	Shepherd	Modified radical vaginal trachelectomy
1998	Maas	Nerve sparing radical hysterectomy
2006	Sert	Robotic radical hysterectomy

Surgical steps for robotic radical hysterectomy:

a) Uterus instrumented with V-care manipulator or a swab on a stick, two vicryl sutures on the cervix and the is closed
b) Folley catheter
c) Veress, pneumoperitoneum, trocars
d) Tredelenburg of 30 degrees
e) 12 mm Hg intra-abdominal pressure
f) Docking and instrumentation
g) Bipolar fenestrated in left arm with bipolar diathermy at 35
h) Scissors in right main port with monopolar diathermy at 35 cut and coagulation Cadier in third arm

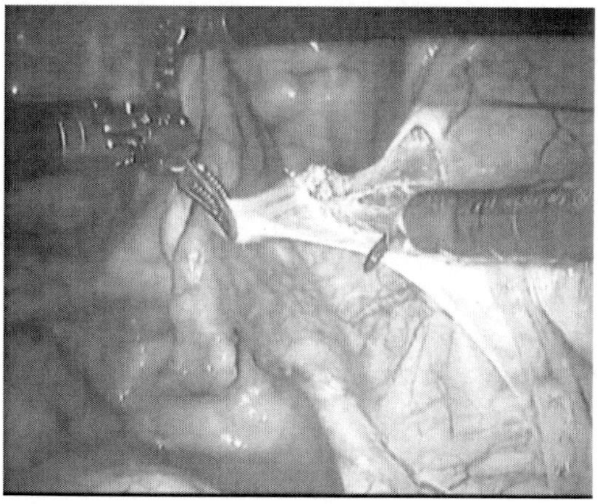

Broads entered.

a) Broads entered after incising with monopolar

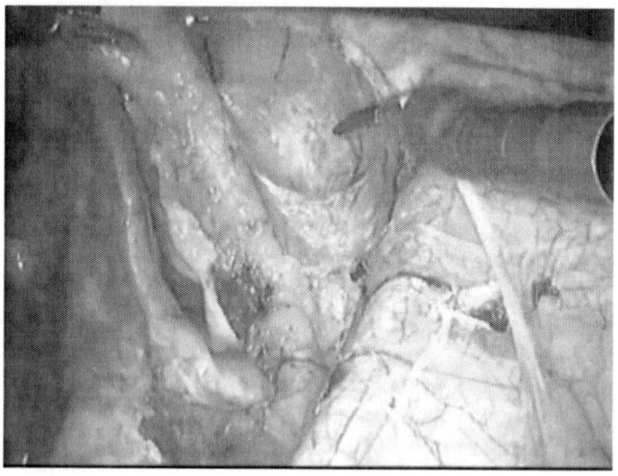

Paravesical and pararectal spaces.

b) Paravesical and pararectal spaces developed to identify cardinals, parametrial web and lateral parametrium

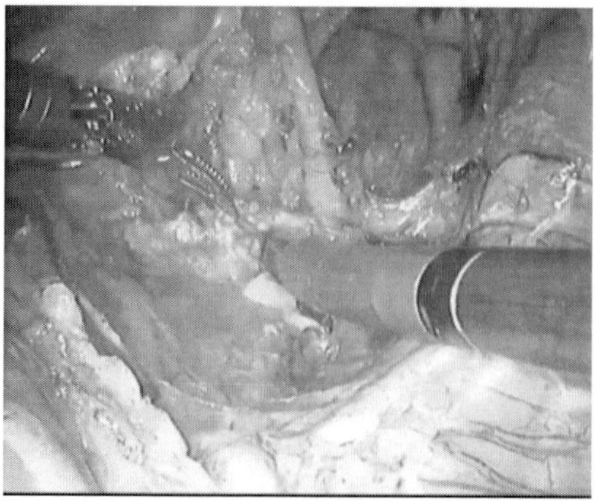

Paravesical and pararectal spaces.

c) Ureters identified bilaterally and traced to the crossing with the uterine arteries
d) Infundibulopelvic ligaments cut with bipolar and monopolar – If adnexae are preserved, the tubo-ovarian pedicles are divided along the lateral wall of the uterus including the broad ligament

Dissection of:

- External iliac nodes from the bifurcation of the common iliac vessels to the inguinal ligament

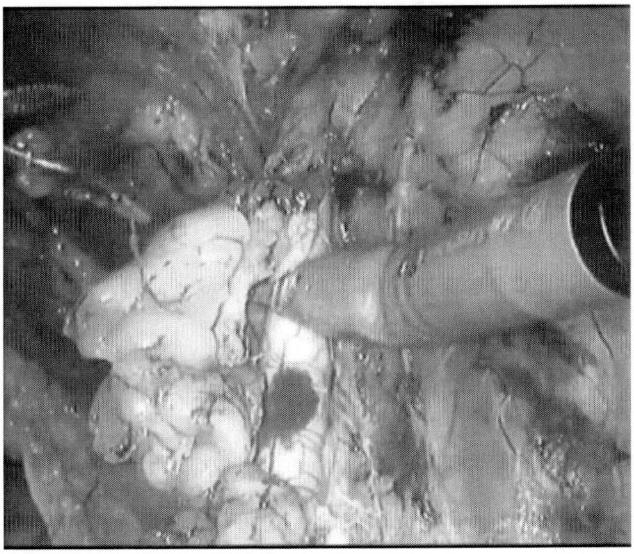

External iliac nodes.

- Obturator nodes above and below the obturator nerve

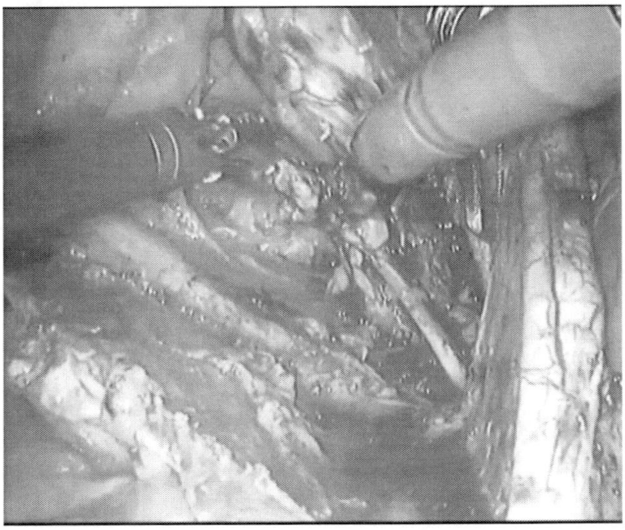

Obturator nodes.

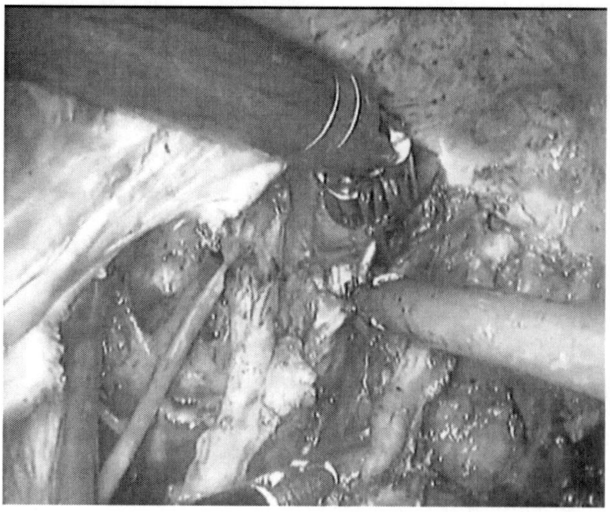

Obturator nodes.

- Ventral and lateral nodes of the hypogastric artery
- Ventral and lateral common iliac nodes from the bifurcation of the common iliacs to the bifurcation of the aorta

In case of positive pelvic lymph nodes, paraaortic lympadenectomy could be performed up to inferior mesenteric artery or to the renal vessels

a) Parametrial division at the origin of the vessels from the internal iliac artery and vein to the level of the deep uterine vein in order to preserve the parasympathetic nerves from S2, S3, S4.

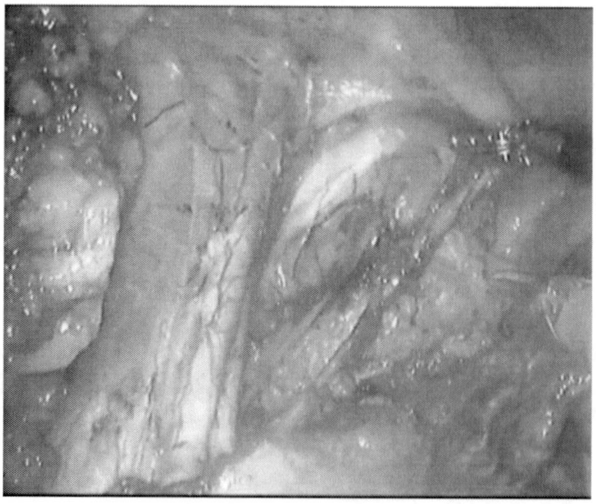

Lymph node dissection.

b) Rectovaginal space developed caudally to the upper vaginal third, ureters separated from peritoneal attachments, uterosacral ligaments dissection at the anterior rectal wall

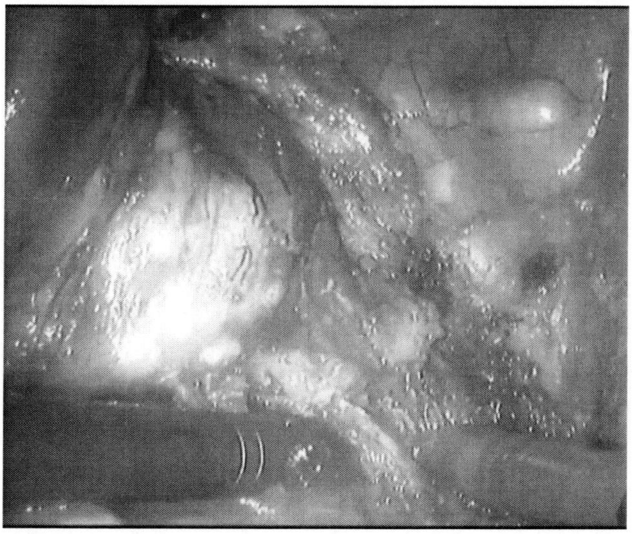

Parametrium.

c) UV fold peritoneum divided with monopolar
d) Bladder reflection to the upper vaginal third
e) Ureter followed to the entrance in the parametrial tunnel
f) A space is created above the ureter with the monopolar and the ventral part of the vesicouterine ligament is transected and the ureter is unroofed and the entrance to the bladder is identified
g) Suspension of ureters, division of paravaginal tissues

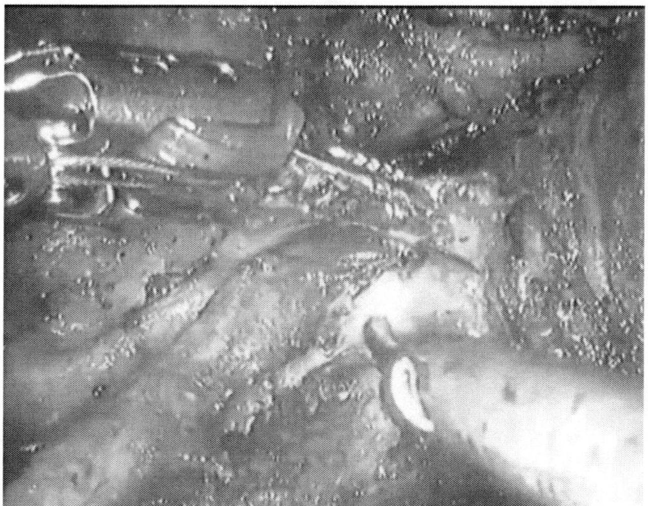

Parametrium.

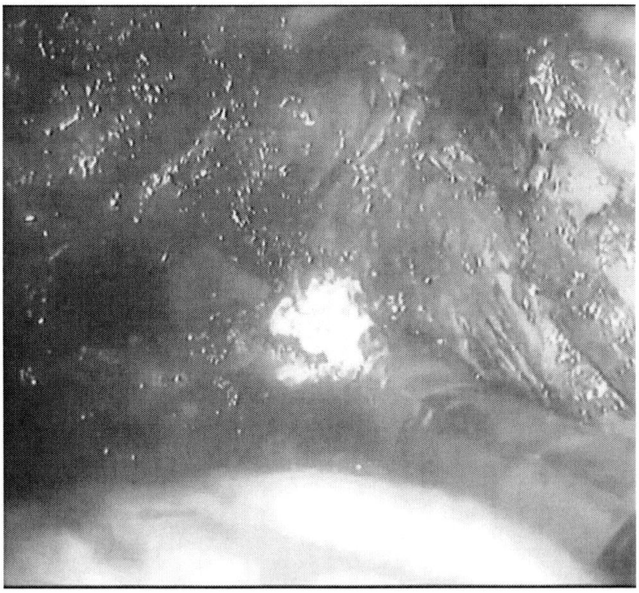

Colpotomy.

h) Vagina entered anteriorly on top of the manipulator and dissection continued circumferentially with monopolar

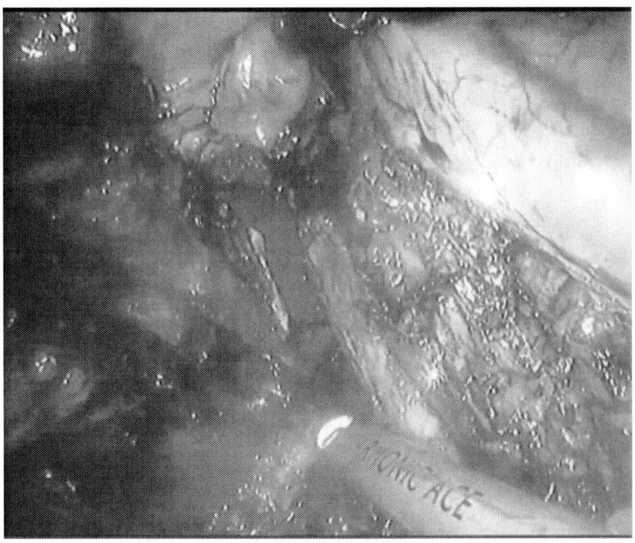

Colpotomy.

i) Specimens extracted through the vagina
j) Glove with swab inserted in vagina to maintain pneumoperitoneum
k) Vaginal vault closed with continuous V-lock, no knot at the end

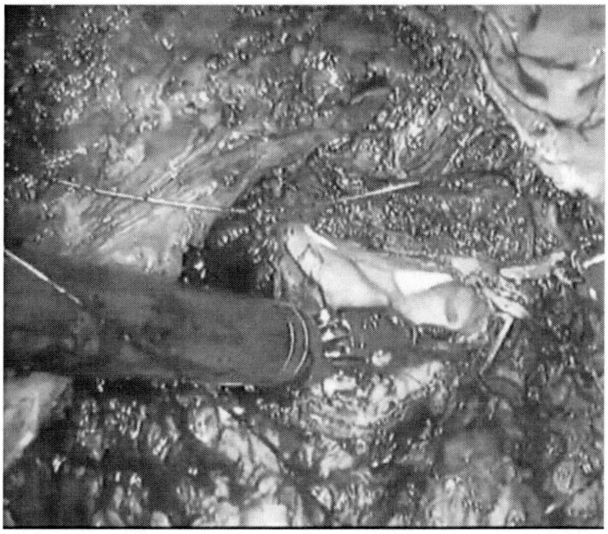

Vaginal vault closure.

l) Haemostasis
m) Undocking

Chapter 19

Surgical Steps for Robotic Radical Trachelectomy

Uterus not instrumented

Swab on a stick in vagina

Folley catheter

Veress, pneumoperitoneum, trocars

Tredelenburg of 30 degrees

12 mm Hg intraabdominal pressure

Docking and instrumentation

Incision over the round ligaments

The peritoneum lateral to infundibulopelvic ligament ligaments is opened bilaterally with ureters identified bilaterally after developing the paravesical and pararectal spaces.

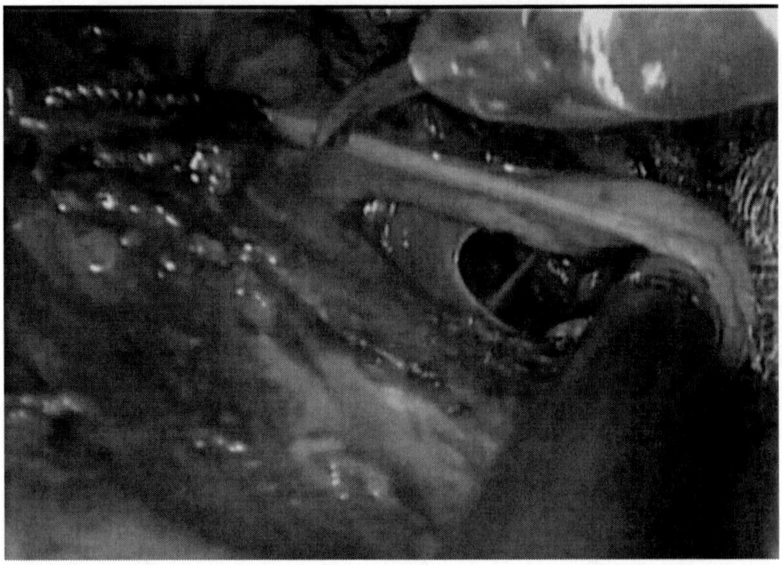

The ureters are dissected from the parametria and mobilized completely to the bladder after division of the anterior and posterior vesicouterine ligaments.

Bladder reflection

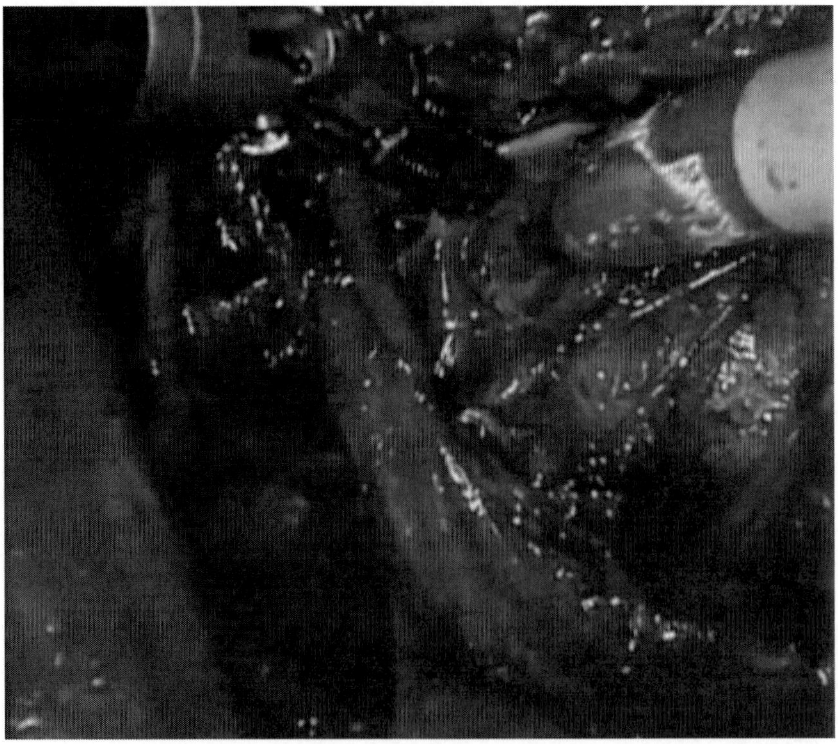

Uterine vessels recognized bilaterally and transected in their origin.

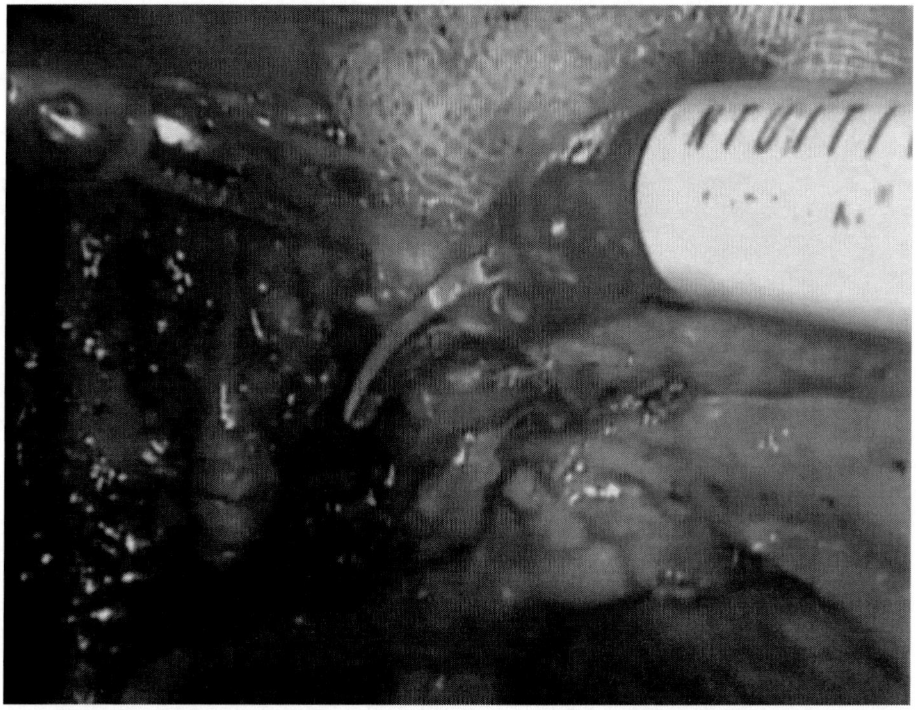

Descending branches of the uterine arteries are recognized and cut.

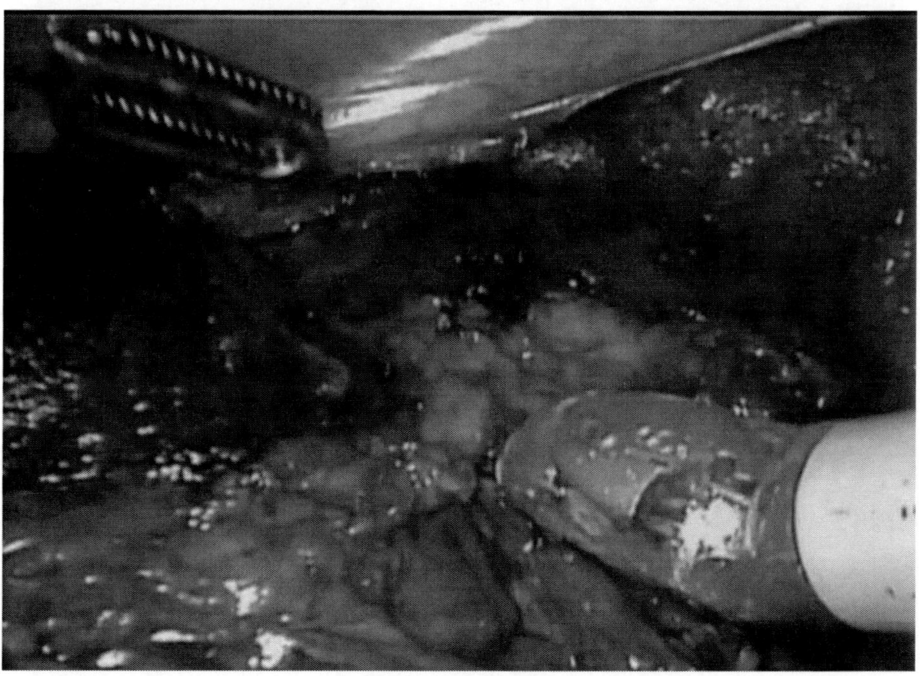

The anterior vesicouterine ligaments are divided.

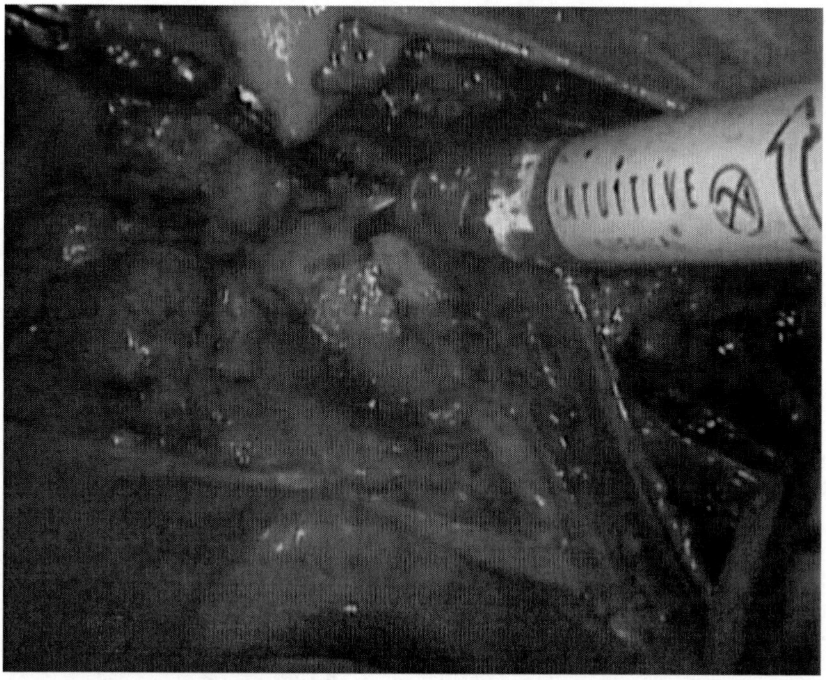

The peritoneum over the rectovaginal space is incised and the uterosacral ligaments cut.

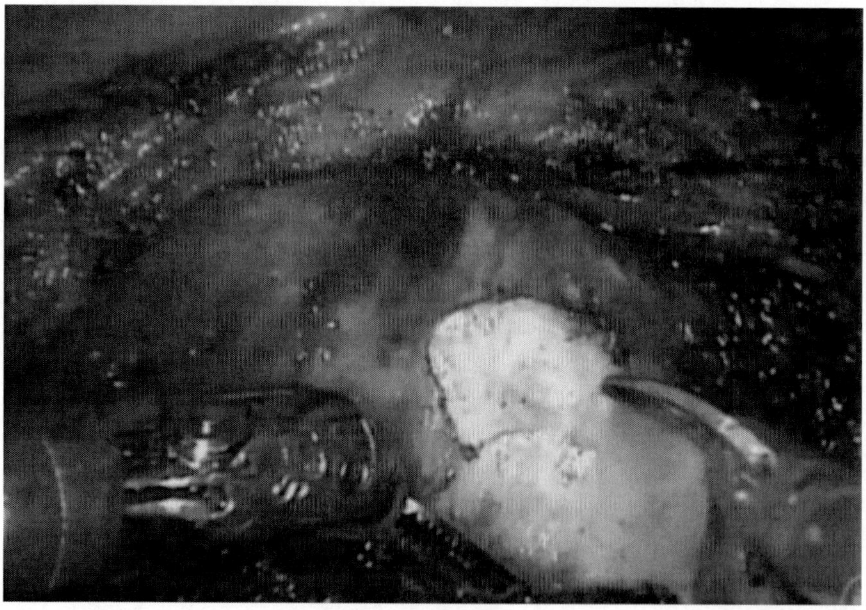

A circumferential incision is made 2 cm below the vaginal stump and excision of cervix at the junction with the uterine body is following.

The specimen including parametria, cervix and vaginal margin is removed vaginally and sent for frozen section in order to clarify if it is at least 1 cm tumor free from the margins.

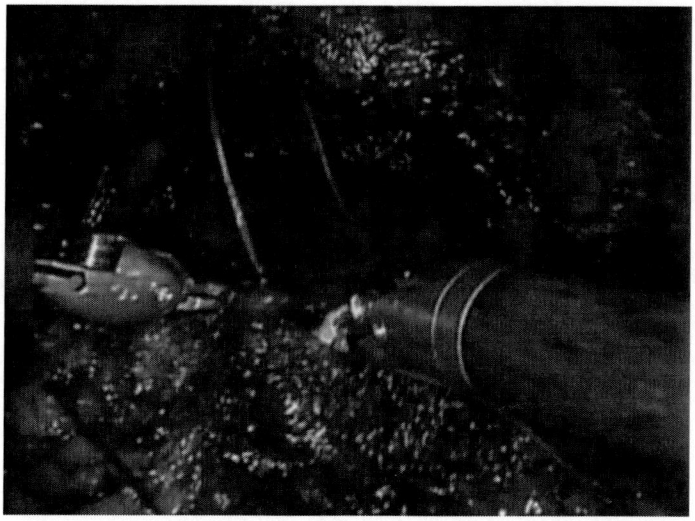

Prolene 0 cerclage suture is applied around cervix with the knot posteriorly.

Free vaginal edges approximated to the uterine edges with interrupted vicryl sutures.

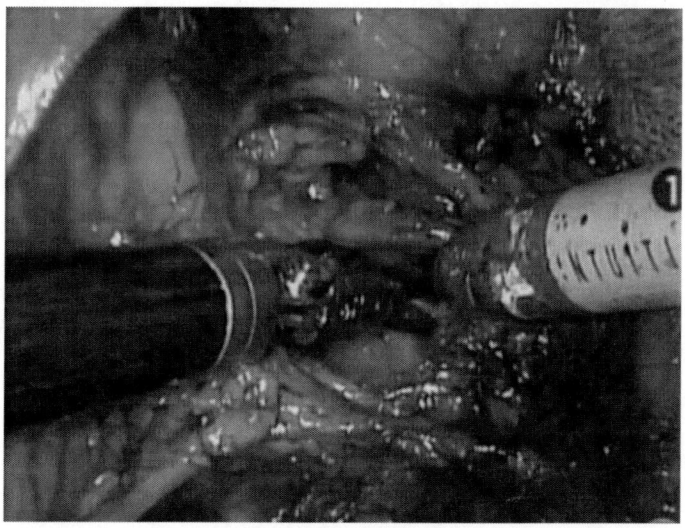

Bilateral pelvic lymphadenectomy is completed from the level of the mid-common iliac vessels to the circumflex iliac vein distally.

Haemostasis
Undocking

Advantages of robotic approach:

- three-dimensional (3D) view
- wrist-like motion of the robotic arms lower blood loss (even < 50 ml)
- higher lymph node retrieval

- fewer wound complications
- fewer urinary tract injuries
- minimal rates of conversion to open
- ideal for obese patients
- reduced length of hospital stay (around 24 hours)
- faster return to normal activities

    - operative time: 144-323 minutes
    - blood loss: 78-165 ml

Possible complications:

- cystotomy
- ureteric injury
- bowel injury

Disadvantages:

- Cost
- Learning curve (operative time continues to decrease with increased experience)

Prognosis:

- The prognosis is related to the stage of the cancer. After proper treatment, the survival rate in 5 year period is up to 93% and up to 63% for women with stage Ia and stage IIa cancer, respectively. The 5 years survival rates decrease to 30% for women with stage III cancer and drops off 15% in patients with stage IV at the time of diagnosis

Chapter 20

Surgical Steps for Robotic Pelvic Lymph Node Sampling/Dissection

a) 2 vicryl sutures on the cervix.
b) Uterus instrumented with UPS manipulator but balloon not inflated and cervical cap tied with the sutures.
c) Indwelling foley at outset.
d) Veress, pneumo and trocars.
e) Side docking. Instrumentation.
f) Bipolar diathermy at 40. Scissors in right main port with monopolar diathermy at 40 cut and coag. Cadiere or Maryland in 3rd arm.
g) Broads entered after incising with monopolar.
h) Ureters identified on both sides.
i) Pelvic side wall entered overlying the external iliac vessels.
j) Uncomplicated and thorough dissection of lymph nodes from the external iliac vessels up to the bifurcation of the common iliac vessels

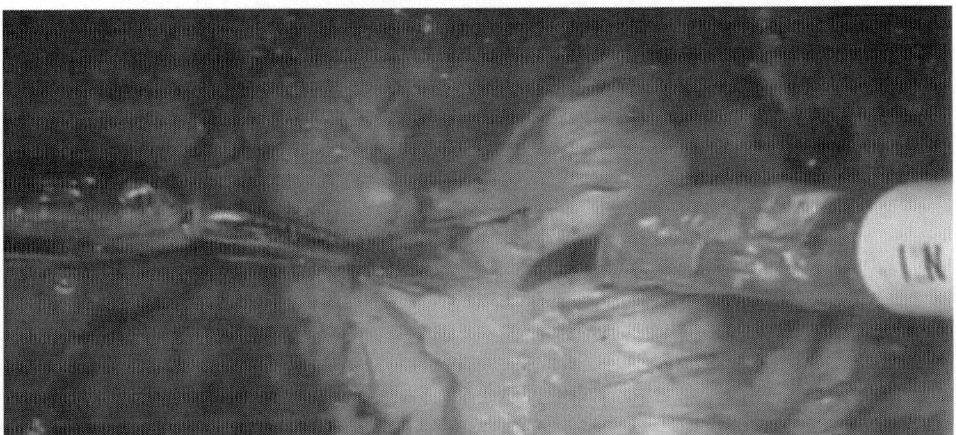

Pelvic lymph node dissection.

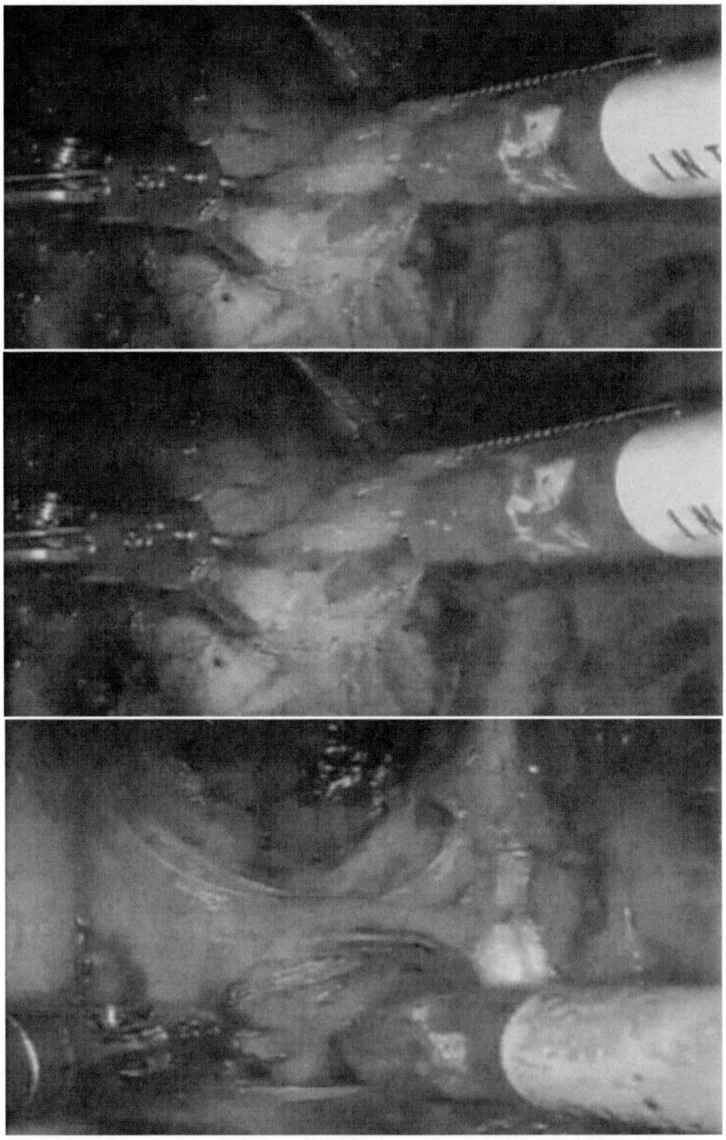

Pelvic lymph node dissection.

h) Internal iliac nodes dissection bilaterally

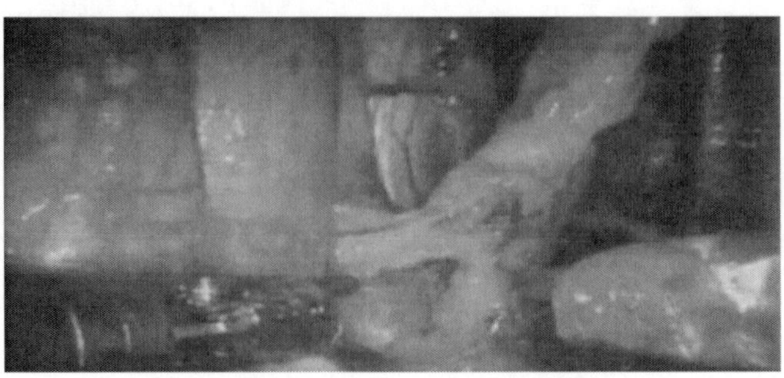

Pelvic lymph node dissection.

i) Boundaries of pelvic lymph node dissection:
- Lateral: genitofemoral nerve
- Medial: ureter
- Inferior: deep iliac circumflex vein

Superior: inferior mesenteric artery

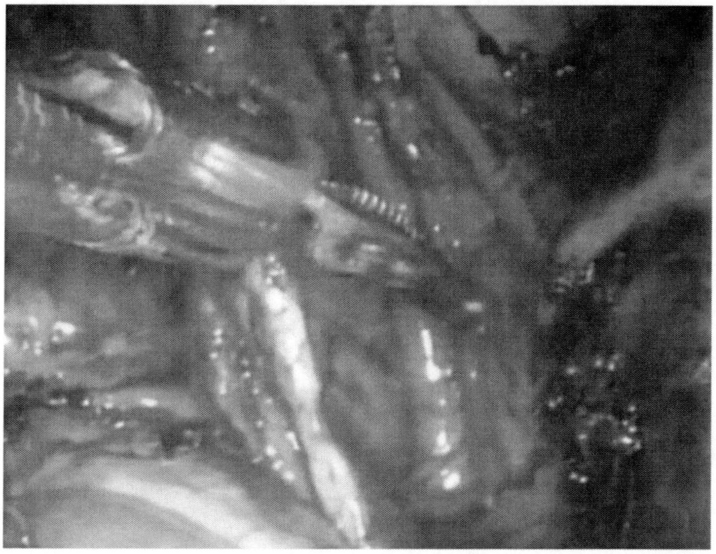

Pelvic lymph node dissection.

j) Recognition of obturator nerve
k) Pelvic lymph nodes extracted through the port in laparoscopic bags.
l) Pelvis washed out.
m) Haemostasis confirmed.
n) Uncomplicated undocking

Chapter 21

The Role of Sentinel Lymph Node in the Robotic Management of Gynecological Cancer

Introduction

The sentinel lymph node (SLN) concept is based on the assumption that all spread from tumors goes through one or several primary draining lymph nodes. If this/these are tumor free, all other nodes should be disease free. Therefore a non-metastatic SLN may allow the removal of only this lymph node. The SLN approach reduces complications caused by the lymphadenectomy but still allows staging of the tumor. The role of SLN biopsy is to preserve control of regional disease, succeed lymph node staging, and avoid excess morbidity.

Cervical Cancer

In surgically treated patients with early cervical cancer, LN metastasis is the most important risk factor for recurrence and death. Accurate knowledge of LN status is essential to tailor adjuvant treatment.

Complete retroperitoneal lymphadenectomy is associated with short- and long-term morbidities such as prolonged duration of surgery, increased blood loss, infection, nerve injury, lymphocyst formation, vascular injury, venous thromboembolism, and lower extremity lymphedema. In operable stage IB1 cervical cancer, prevalence of LN metastasis is estimated to be about 15%. This suggests that up to 85% of these patients may undergo lymphadenectomy for no direct benefit while being subjected to the potential risk of associated morbidities.

Endometrial Cancer

Endometrial cancer is the most common cancer of the female genital tract. Most cases of endometrial cancer are diagnosed in stage I with a fairly good prognosis. The presence of lymph node metastases has a major impact in the prognosis of patients with the disease.

Surgical staging is part of the initial treatment algorithm. The surgical management of endometrial cancer includes peritoneal cytology, total hysterectomy with bilateral adnexectomy, and lymph node sampling (pelvic and paraaortic lymphadenectomy) to assess lymph node status. Lymphadenectomy allows precise determination of prognosis, accurate tailoring of adjuvant treatment, and could lead to a small survival advantage. More specifically, the 5-year disease free survival in patients with negative lymph nodes has been reported to be 90% compared to 54% for those with positive lymph nodes.

However, women with endometrial cancer usually suffer from commorbidity related to their age, obesity, diabetes mellitus and hypertension facts that should be considered in the management plan. More specifically, routine lymphadenectomy adds an extra 30 minutes surgical time and it is associated with an increased risk of intra- or postoperative complications. It is also known that about 8 in 10 women with stage I endometrial cancer do not have any pelvic lymph node metastases. For this reason, it is suggested that lymphadenectomy could be omitted in women with endometrioid cancer and no myometrial invasion (independently of grade or tumour size) and in those with grade 1-2 tumours, myometrial invasion below 50%, tumour diameter below 2 cm and no evidence of tumour outside the corpus.

Lymphatic drainage of the uterus is complex including the obturator, iliac (external, internal, and common), caval and aortic vessels, the parametrial tissue and the presacral space. Three routes for lymphatic drainage exist: via the hypogastric or obturator regions to the common iliac lymph nodes, along the round ligaments to reach inguinal lymph nodes, and via the ovarian vessels to the paraaortic lymph nodes. Isolated paraaortic lymph node involvement without pelvic lymph node involvement is only detected in 1-3% of patients with endometrial cancer.

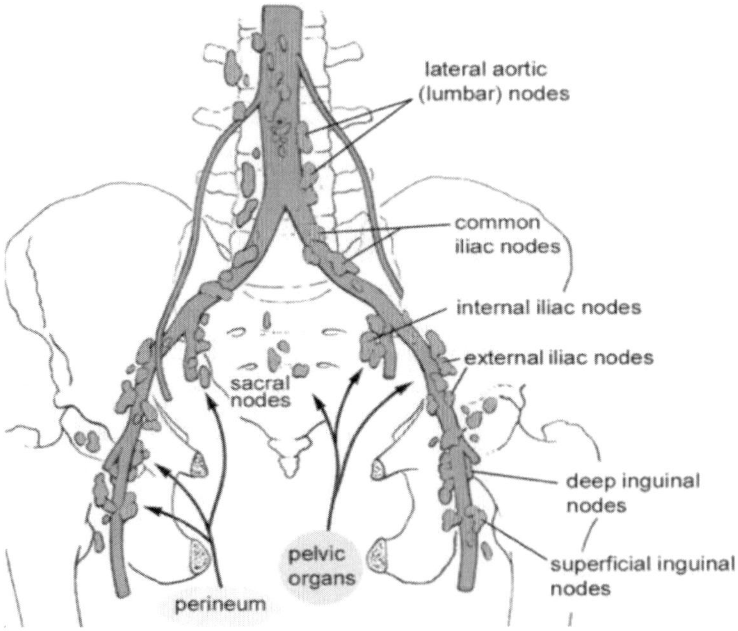

Main lymph nodes related to the pelvic organs.

Till now the SLN concept is used in some prospective studies.

Method

Lymphatic mapping of pelvic sentinel lymph nodes using fluorescence near-infrared imaging of indocyanine green (ICG) and colorimetric imaging of isosulfan blue (ISB) dyes:

a) One mL ISB is injected submucosally in four quadrants of the cervix.
a) 0.5 mL ICG [1.25mg/mL] injected immediately.
b) Placement of a uterine manipulator.
c) Retroperitoneal spaces are dissected for colorimetric detection of lymphatic pathways.
d) The da Vinci® camera is switched to fluorescence imaging and results recorded.
e) SLNs are removed for permanent analysis with ultra-sectioning, H&E, and IHC staining.
f) Robotic hysterectomy and adnexectomy is performed followed by a complete pelvic lymphadenectomy +/- paraaortic lymphadenectomy if the general state of the patient is considered to be sufficient by the gynecologist.

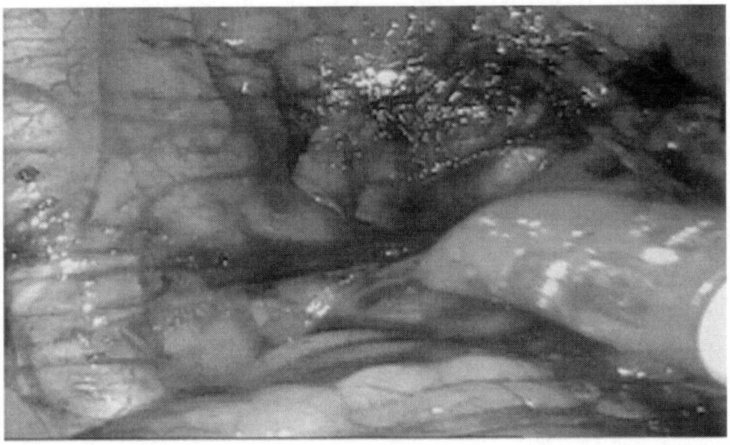

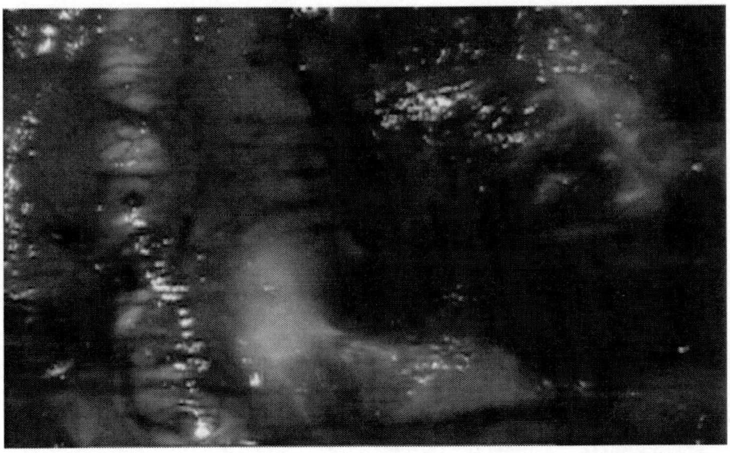

Sentinel lymph node.

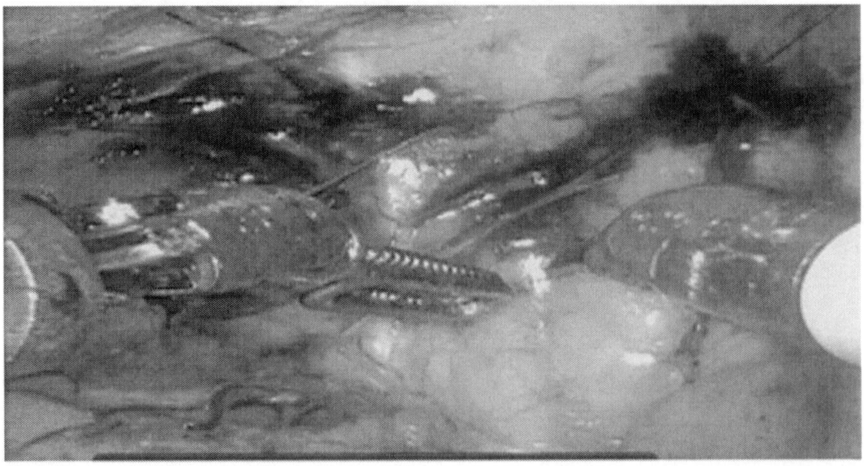

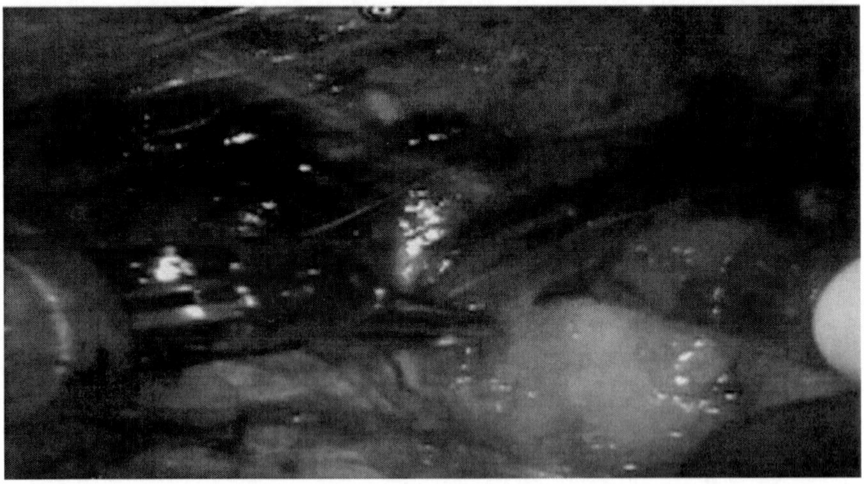

Sentinel lymph node.

Sentinel lymph nodes are sent to pathological examination separately from the lymph node-bearing tissue of the pelvic and paraaortic regions.

All sentinel lymph nodes are cut perpendicular to their long axis into 3- to 4-mm sections and submitted for routine hematoxylin and eosine staining (H and E). Hematoxylin and eosin negative sections are going to be examined by immunohistochemistry with an anticytokeratin antibody. Sentinel lymph nodes are considered positive for tumor involvement when they contain macro- or micrometastases. The size of lymph node metastases is estimated with an eye-piece micrometer. Micrometastasis is a single focus of metastatic disease measuring less than 2 mm in a given node.

Chapter 22

Nerve-Sparing Technique in Robotic Assisted Gynaecological Surgery

Nerve-sparing technique at a radical hysterectomy has been proposed as a procedure that improves the quality of life by reducing urinary, rectal and sexual dysfunctions. Even though, there is no apparent consensus about which parts of the uterine ligaments can be spared during this procedure, the preservation of pelvic autonomic nerves is the key for the maintenance of the control of bladder, the rectal functions and for sexual arousal.

Technique

b) Low lithotomy position with the legs in Allen stirrups is the preferred position of the patient. The arms are tucked laterally at the patient's sides. The monitor as well as the tower with the electrosurgical generators is placed on the left side of the patient.
c) Foley catheter and uterine manipulator are placed.
d) Umbilical incision with Veress needle or open Hasson approach.
e) With the use of a 12 mm supra-umbilical trocar, the laparoscope arm is inserted in the abdominal cavity while three 8 mm trocars are also inserted. The 8 mm trocars are positioned under direct visualization in both iliac fossae and at the midline between the umbilicus and the right subcostal margin. A 10 mm trocar is also placed between the umbilicus and the left subcostal margin, along the midline. Insufflation of CO_2 (up to 12 mmHg) into the abdominal cavity for the creation of pneumoperitoneum is succeeded through insufflation cannulae.
f) The patient then is placed in a Trendelenburg position (in 30–35°). The da Vinci robot is docked between the legs or at the right side.
g) The uterus and the ovaries are inspected. Both the round ligament and the infundibulopelvic ligament are coagulated and cut. Retroperitoneal space is opened to identify the ureter, medially to the resected infundibulopelvic ligament The peritoneum overlying the ureter is also resected. The ureter is removed laterally, the hypogastric nerve is identified posterior and medially to the ureter. Keeping always

the ureter and the hypogastric nerve under vision, we extend the peritoneal cut to the pouch of Douglas. The rectum is dissected from the posterior part of the vaginal wall till we reach the elevator muscle of anus.

h) With a Cadiere grasper, pararectal space is dissected until the level of uterine veins, preserving the branches of the pelvic splachnic nerves. When the uterine vessels are identified is coagulated and ligated. Dissection is continued caudally in the plane, anterior to the dissected uterine arteries. Posterior to this paravesical area, the cardinal and the uterosacral ligament are identified and cut, sparing the hypogastric nerves that lie lateral to the uterosacral ligaments. Underneath the dissected uterine veins, there are the branches of pelvic splachnic nerves, which direct in the direction of the inferior hypogastric plexus.

i) Remaining constantly medial to the hypogastric nerve the dissection is continued by selectively cut some branches of the hypogastric nerve and the inferior hypogastric plexus which are recognized in the connective tissue immediately posteriolaterally to the vagina. This completes the posterior part of the dissection. The important at this stage of the procedure is to preserve intact the bladder branch of the inferior hypogastric plexus and to move aside the nerve plane and the homolateral ureter.

j) Peritoneum, from one to the other round ligament, is dissected. Also, peritoneum is cut between the infundibulopelvic ligament and the round ligament in order to make visible the majority of ureter. With a Maryland forceps is dissected the ureteric tunnel. All the veins through the roof of the ureteric tunnel are identified, ligated and cut while the ureter is pushed laterally.

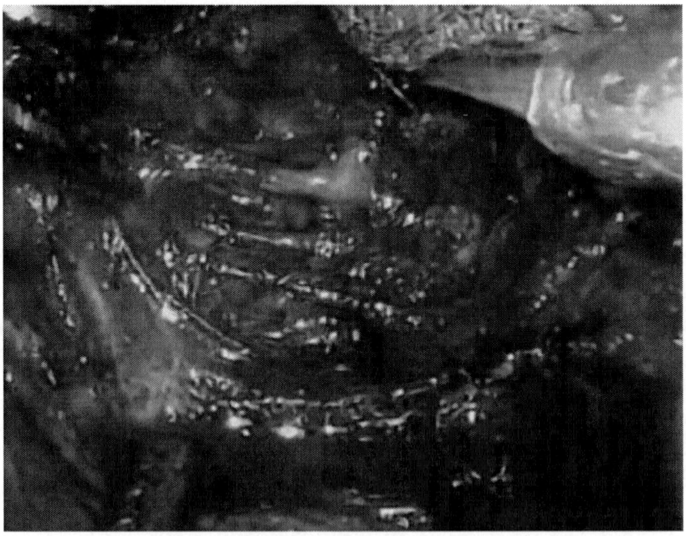

Nerve plexus.

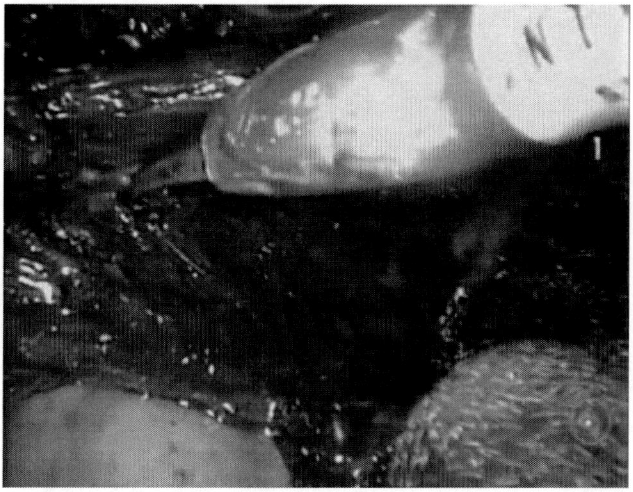

Nerve plexus.

k) The movement of the ureter at the same time also moves both the ureteric and the bladder branches of the inferior hypogastric plexus laterally at the same side. The posterior side of the vesicouterine ligament also contains veins of bladder which are clipped and cut. The bladder branch that passes under the inferior vesical vein can be visible and preserved. The uterine and inferiorly the cervical branches of the inferior hypogastric plexus are selectively cut at their anterior part.
l) Bladder dissection - colpotomy.
m) Uterus and adnexae are removed through the vaginal canal. The vaginal cuff is closed with interrupted sutures, in preference with barbed ones.
n) In case it is necessary to proceed to pelvic lymphadenectomy, all the excised lymph nodes are placed in endobags.

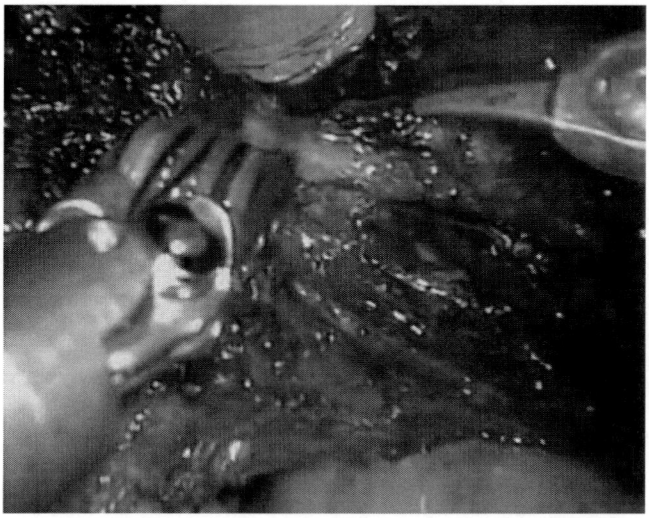

Vesical branch of inferior hypogastric plexus (IHP).

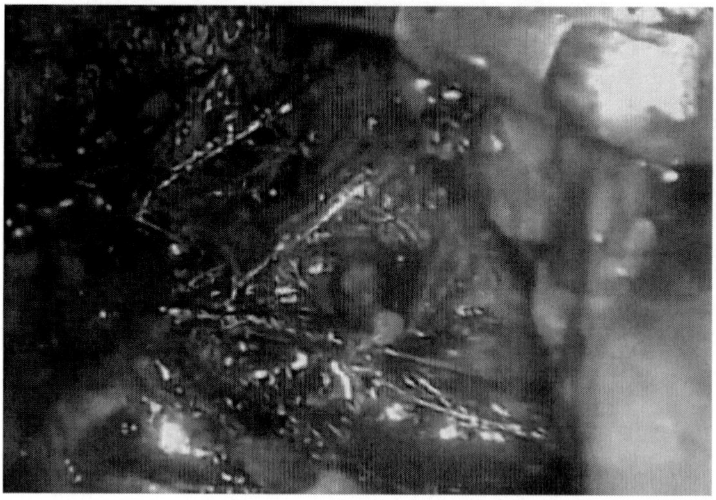

Inferior hypogastric plexus.

Chapter 23

Robotic Pelvic Exenteration in Cervical Cancer

- cervical cancer is the second most common type of neoplasia in premenopausal women
- pelvic exenteration is defined as the en-bloc resection of internal reproductive organs, bladder, pelvic ureters, rectum, sigmoid colon along with the pelvic peritoneum and the loco regional lymph nodes.
- the pelvic exenteration can be an indication in cases of primary or secondary surgical therapy in order to treat or to offer a palliative treatment in patients who present with the following criteria:
  a) Absence of distant metastasis
  b) Tumor with diameter <30mm
  c) Absence of any adherence to the pelvic side wall
  d) More than one year relapse time

Indications for the performance of pelvic exenteration

- in cases of disabling urinary symptoms (urgency, urinary incontinence and nocturia)
- faecal incontinence or bowel obstruction
- urinary obstructions not responding to drainage procedures
- debilitating pelvic pain
- presence of fistulas in pelvis
- recurrent haemorrhage
- recurrent pelvic sepsis

Contraindications for the performance of pelvic exenteration

- the presence of major medical and psychiatric pathologies
- extrapelvic disease associated with poor prognosis
- immobile tumors fixed to the pelvic sidewalls

- the presence of tumor invasion of the proximal lumbosacral spine (S1 or higher)
- tumor invasion of lumbosacral plexus/sciatic nerves or the external or common iliac vessels
- lymphoedema to the lower extremities

Advantages of the robotic assisted treatment

- robotic systems offer the possibility to dissect down and into the narrow pelvic floor
- three-dimension stereoscopic vision by the use of binocular optics
- filtration of the surgeon's tremor
- less fatigue for the operator
- a wide range of motions is permitted by the utilization of articulated instruments, increasing the ability of the operator to work in restricted spaces of the pelvic floor.
- the use of harmonic scalpel consents the control of the pelvic vessels and the transection of the ligamentous attachments around the extirpated pelvic structures
- the 360° motion of the robotic wrist allows the fine sewing necessary in the ureteral ileostomy and in the ileal loop urinary diversion
- the minimally invasive characteristics of the robotic assisted technique can offer less blood loss, less pain, better aesthetic result, shorter recovery
- quicker return to normal activity mean that postoperative treatment (either chemotherapy or radiation) can begin earlier

Disadvantages of the robotic assisted treatment

- high costs of robotic technology
- bulky machinery and the necessity for staff specific training
- in case of local invasion of the pelvic ureters, the performance of urinary diversion can be accomplished either with mini laparotomy or with hand-assisted technique

Table. Characteristics of studies regarding robotic pelvic exenteration in cases of cervical cancer

First author, year, country	Publication type	Age of patient (in years)	Histological type	Stage of primary neoplasia*	Type of operation performed	Duration of the procedure (in min)	Blood loss (in ml)	Complications§	Post-operative stay (in days)	Follow up
Jauffret, 2011, France	case series	67	squamous cell	NR	anterior pelvic exenteration / lymphadenectomy	480	200	-	median (range): 6 (3-24)	23 mo
		59	squamous cell	NR	anterior pelvic exenteration	480	400	-		31 mo
Davis, 2010, USA	case report	50	squamous cell	IVA	anterior pelvic exenteration: 2 pts (12mm), 3 pts (8mm)	mean: 540	mean: 550	NR	8	NR
		58	NR	NR†				NR		NR
Lambaudie, 2010, France	case report	65	squamous cell	IB2	anterior pelvic exenteration: 5 pts	480	200	perineal abscess Miami's stoma fistula	53	12 mo
		60		IIB		480	400	ureteral stenosis	25	8 mo
		43		NR		600	500	-	30	2 mo
Lim, 2009, USA	case report	57	squamous cell	IVA	total pelvic exenteration: 5 pts	375	375	-	10	NR

Abbreviations: NR = not referred, pts = ports, mo = months, VAIN = vaginal intraepithelial neoplasia.
*According to FIGO classification.
§Related to robotic pelvic exenteration.
†Locally advanced cervical cancer.

Chapter 24

The Role of Robot in Ovarian Cancer

Incidence:

- the fifth most common neoplasia in female population
- estimated lifetime risk is almost 1.6%, while women with affected first-degree relatives present a 5% lifetime risk

Symptoms:

- asymptomatic (common finding changes in bowel or urinary habits) – "silent killer"
- the suspicion is posed in elderly patients with ascites, combined with fixed, rapid growing tumor.

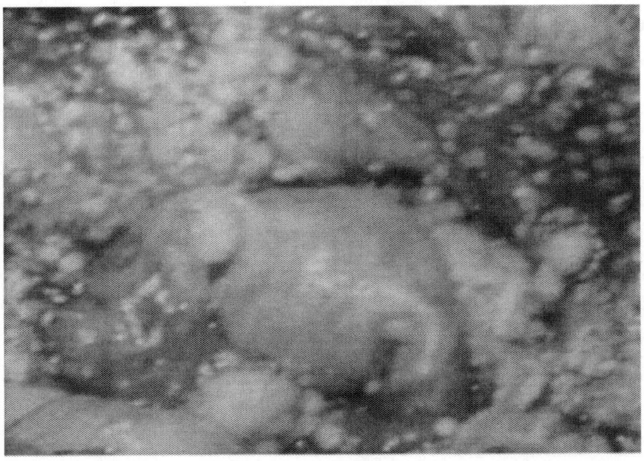

Ovarian cancer.

Diagnosis:

- Usually, it is diagnosed in late stages.
- raised CA-125 levels or CA19-9 in cases of mucinous tumors and transvaginal ultrasound
- U/S: solid or mixed cystic tumor may be present

Preoperative evaluation:

- clinical and gynecological examination
- transvaginal ultrasound
- CT chest-abdomen-pelvis
- MRI abdomen-pelvis
- PET/CT

Histology:

- Adenocarcinoma (89.7%)
- Serous, mucinous, endometrioid, clear cell, transitional

2014 FIGO ovarian, fallopian tube, and peritoneal cancer staging system and corresponding TNM:

Stage	
I	Tumor is limited to the ovaries or to the fallopian tube.
Ia	The lesion is confined inside to one ovary.
Ib	The lesion is confined inside both ovaries.
Ic	Tumor located in one or both ovaries, with surface infiltration of an ovary or with presence of tumor cells in peritoneal lavage or with ovary ruptures before or during surgical operation.
II	The lesion expands to one or both ovaries or fallopian tubes with pelvic extension.
IIa	Presence of tumor lesions implanted at uterus and/or the fallopian tubes and/or ovaries.
IIb	Extension of tumor to another organ in the pelvis (always limited in pelvis).
III	Tumor is extended outside pelvis but limited into the peritoneal cavity.
IIIa	Microscopic peritoneal metastasis beyond the pelvis (no macroscopic tumor).
IIIb	Macroscopic peritoneal metastasis beyond the pelvis2 cm or less in greatest dimension.
IIIc	Macroscopic peritoneal metastasis beyond the pelvis>2 cm in greatest dimension and/or regional lymph node metastasis (presence of tumour to capsule of liver and spleen without parenchymal involvement).
IV	Presence of distant lesions beyond the peritoneal cavity.
IVa	Parenchymal lesions or pleural effusion with tumor cells.
IVb	Presence of metastases to extra-abdominal organs.

Surgical management:

- Minimally invasive surgical technique is safe and effective in borderline ovarian tumors and early ovarian cancer
- No sufficient evidence to support its use in advanced disease
  - Concerns regarding:
  - tumor rupture
  - port site metastasis
- adequate abdominal exploration & staging
- In cases of low stage tumors, well-differentiated and limited to the ovary, surgical treatment may be sufficient
- The type of operation depends on the tumor stage at the diagnosis and at the histology of the lesion. In case of involvement of one ovary or both ovaries can be opted either unilateral salpingo-oophorectomy or bilateral salpingo-oophorectomy. In stage II or higher, complete open debulking is advised

Advantages of robotic approach:

- three-dimensional (3D) view
- wrist-like motion of the robotic arms lower blood loss (even < 50 ml)
- higher lymph node retrieval
- fewer wound complications
- fewer urinary tract injuries
- minimal rates of conversion to open
- ideal for obese patients
- reduced length of hospital stay (around 24 hours)
- faster return to normal activities

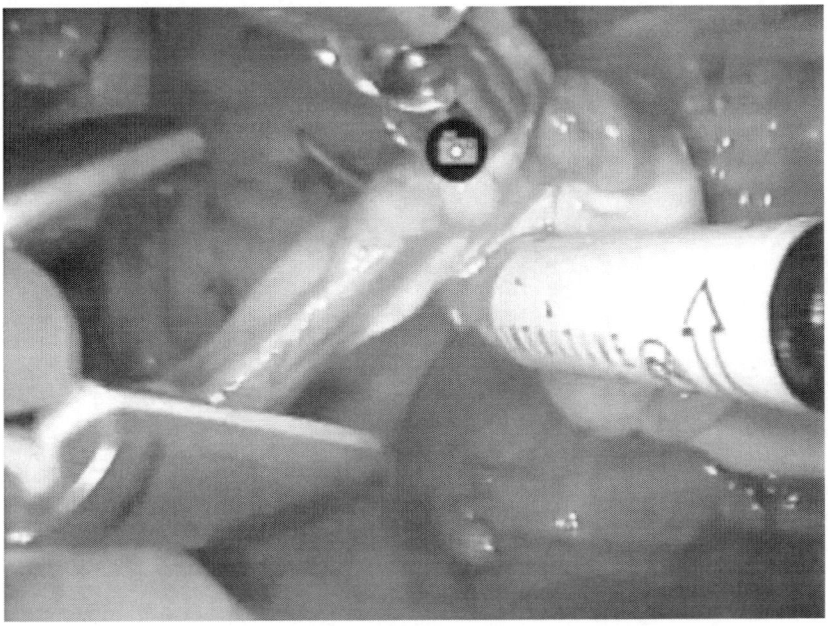

Salpingo-oophorectomy.

Disadvantages:

- Cost
- Learning curve (operative time continues to decrease with increased experience)

Prognosis:

- ovarian cancer is often correlated with poor prognosis
- 5 year survival rate for all stages is almost 40%

Chapter 25

Omentectomy/Omental Biopsy

During supracolic omentectomy, the omentum should be removed from the greater curvature of the stomach and transverse colon. Care must be taken to secure the small omental branches of the right gastric artery. The key anatomical features are the hepatic and splenic flexure of the colon, the spleen and its vascular supply.

After removing the omentum from the hepatic flexure of the transverse colon, the right gastroepiploic artery and its short gastric branches are identified. Small defects are made between each of the short gastric branches in order to ligate them. When the omentum is completely removed from the stomach and the left gastroepiploic artery has been stapled, the remaining omentum is removed from the transverse colon. In case of an omental biopsy, a part of the omentum is excised for diagnostic and staging purposes. Careful haemostasis is essential. The procedure can be performed with side docking and with the use of Maryland/Cadiere, scissors and fenestrated bipolar.

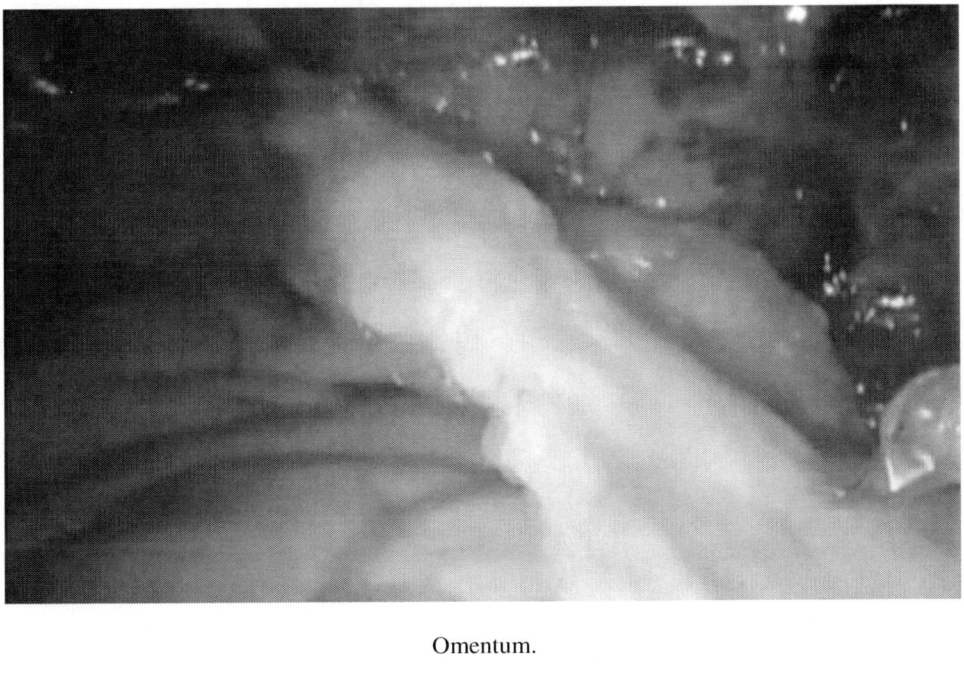

Omentum.

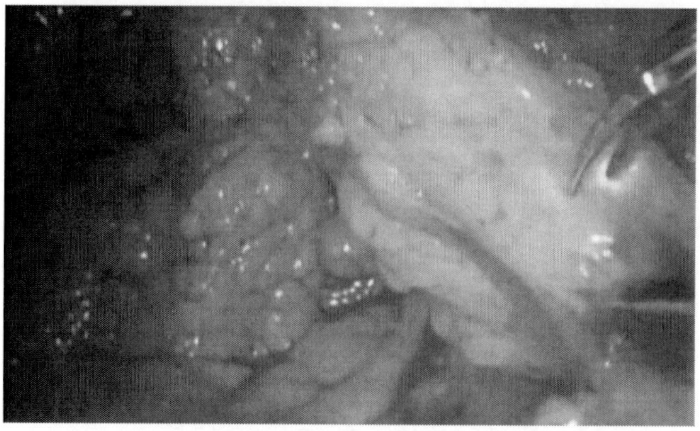

Omentectomy.

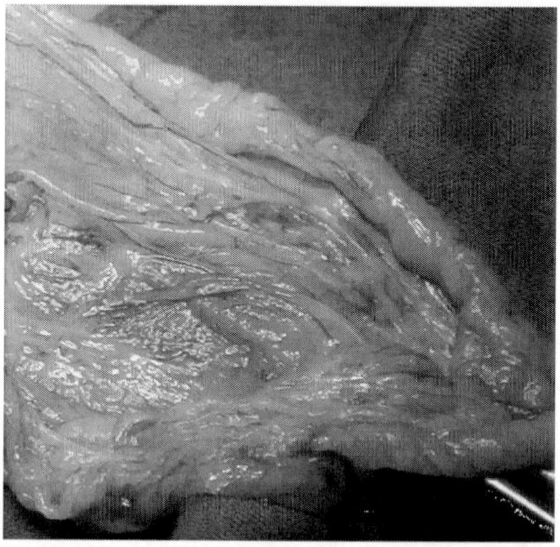

Omentum.

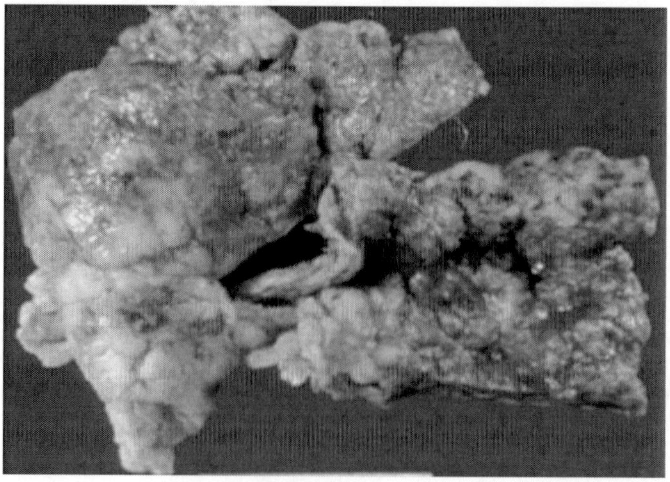

Omentum.

Chapter 26

Appendicectomy

Scissors and fenestrated bipolar are the instruments used. The blood supply for the appendix comes from the appendiceal artery, a branch of the ileocolic artery. The mesoappendix containing the appendiceal artery is divided and ligated down to the serosa of the appendix where it joins the cecum

Two Vicryl ties are used in the appendiceal base at the proposed level of division. The appendiceal stump can be ligated. Careful haemostasis should be achieved. Appendix could be removed through the ports.

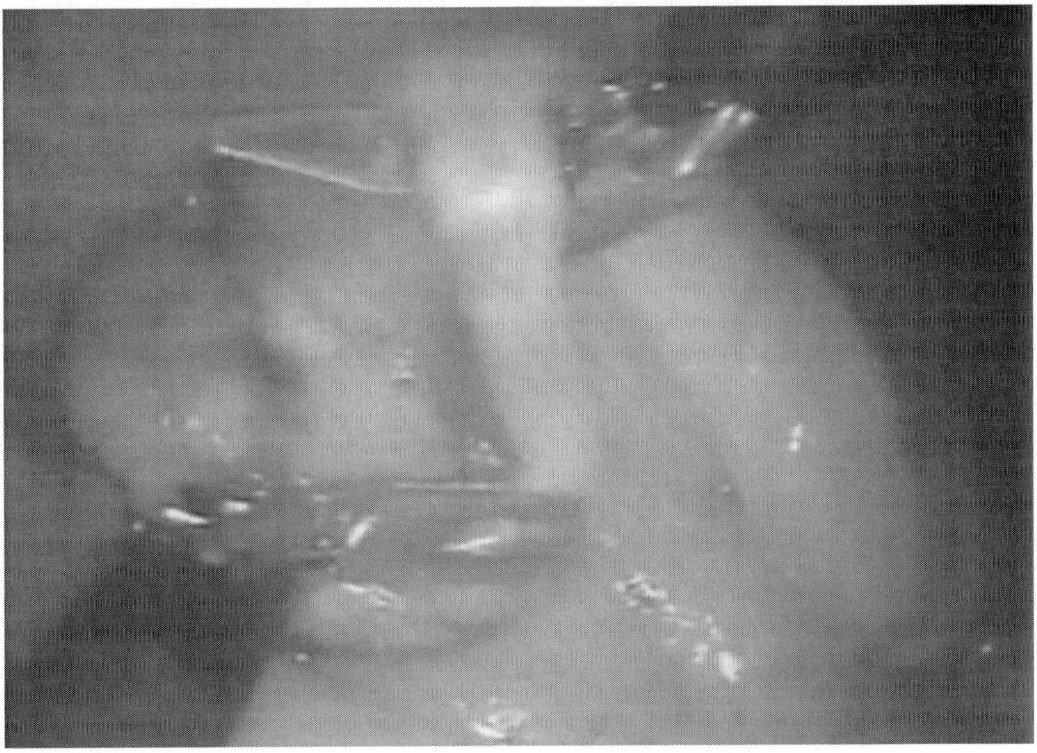

Steps of appendicectomy.

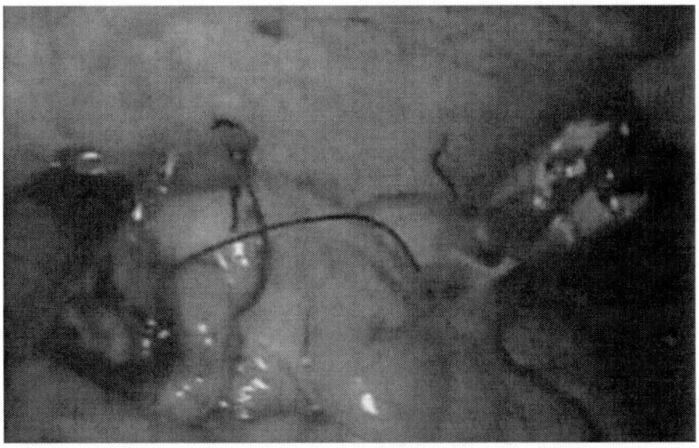

Steps of appendicectomy.

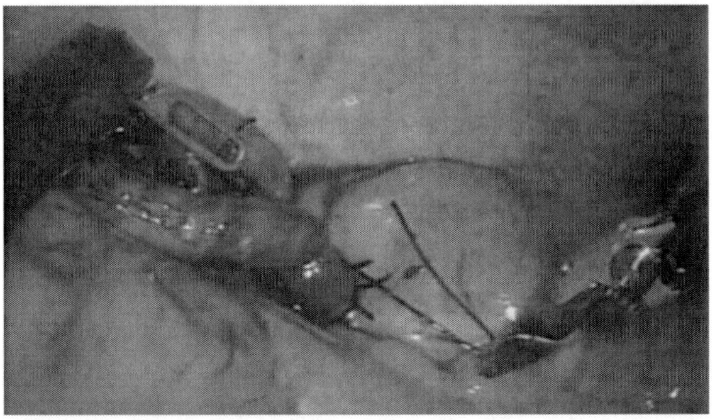

Steps of appendicectomy.

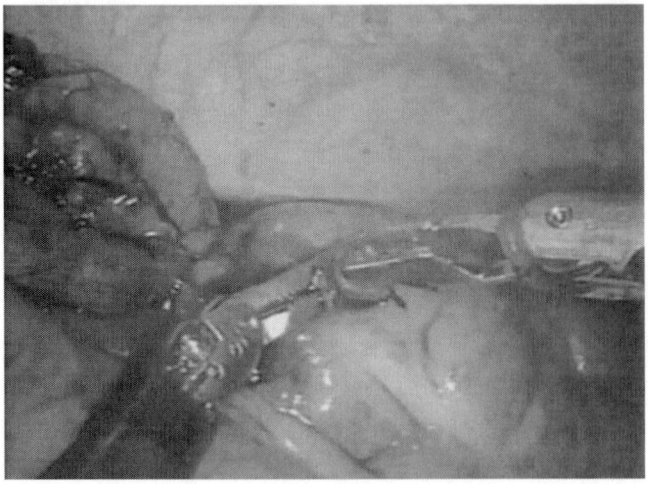

Steps of appendicectomy.

Chapter 27

Robotic versus Laparoscopic versus Abdominal versus Vaginal Hysterectomy

Author/ Year	Operations	Number of patients	Operation time (min)	EBL (ml)	Conversion rate	Intraoperative complications	Hospital stay (days)	Postoperative complications
Payne et al., 2008	RH vs LH	100 vs 100	119 vs 92	61 vs 113	4 vs 9	Cystotomy: 1 vs 2, Enterotomy 0 vs 1	1 vs 1.6	Major: none, minor 1 vs 0
Nezhat et al., 2009	RH vs LH	26 vs 50	276 vs 206	250 vs 300	0 vs 0	none	1 vs 1.05	none
Shashooua et al., 2009	RH vs LH	22 vs 44	142 vs 122	114 vs 99	0 vs 0	none	1 VS 1.4	Cuff dehiscence 0 vs 1, minor: 1 vs 0
Giep et al., 2010	RH vs LAVH-LH	237 vs 265	90 vs 125	59 vs 168	1.7 vs 0.4	Cystotomy 1 vs 1	1 vs 1.2	PEs: 2 vs 1, abcess 1 vs 1, minor: 6 vs 3
Sarlos et al., 2010	RH vs LH	40 vs 40	109 vs 83	50 vs 81	0	0	3.3 vs 3.9	Major: 0, minor 0 vs 5
Matthews et al., 2010	RH vs LH vs VH vs AH	65 vs 21 vs 63 vs 113	NS	82 vs 260 vs 190 vs 430	0 vs 12% vs 3.4%	0	1.5 vs 1.8 vs 1.7 vs 3.5	Major: 4.3% vs 7% vs 11% vs 23%
Kilic et al., 2011	RH vs LH vs VH	25 vs 34 vs 11	286 vs 208 vs 164	137 vs 243 vs 243	8 vs 5.9	Cystotomy 1 vs 1	1.8 vs 2.3 vs 2	Cuff dehiscence: 1 vs 1 vs 0, minor 4 vs 9 vs 3

Table (Continued)

Author/ Year	Operations	Number of patients	Operation time (min)	EBL (ml)	Conversion rate	Intraoperative complications	Hospital stay (days)	Postoperative complications
Geppert et al/2011	RH vs AH	25 vs 64	136 vs 110	100 vs 300	NS	none	1.6 vs 3.8	Cuff dehiscence: 2 vs 0, rectocele 0 vs 1
Soto et al., 2011	RH vs LH	47 vs 77	150.8±33.5 vs 111.45±33.22	<200 32 vs 34 >200 12 vs 37	0 vs 3	0 vs 1	1.9±0.95 vs 2.2±1.14	none
Orady et al., 2012	RH vs LH vs VH vs LAVH	135 vs 46 vs 34 vs 82	median (range): 169 (80–625) vs 194 (103–386) vs 98.5 (29–286) vs 144 (67–398)	median (range): 50 (10–1,000) vs 150 (25–700) vs 150 (50–9,000) vs 250 (75–2,000)	0 vs 1 vs 1 vs 1	Major: 15 vs 6 vs 2 vs 9 Minor: 12 vs 9 vs 10 vs 16	median: 1 vs 1 vs 1 vs 1	NM
Nicole et al., 2012	RH vs LH vs AH	102 vs 115 vs 79	mean (range): 203 (84-396) vs 133 (48-306) vs 132 (51-258)	mean (range): 69 (10-400) vs 86 (10-700) vs 215 (50-2,000)	7 vs 9	NM	mean (range): 1.4 (1-9) vs 1.4 (1-9) vs 3.8 (1-15)	Urinary Tract Infection: 4 vs 1 vs 3 Vaginal Cuff Separation: 1 vs 1 vs 0
								Pulmonary Embolism: 0 vs 0 vs 1 Cystotomy Repair: 0 vs 0 vs 1
								Clostridium Difficile Colitis: 0 vs 0 vs 1 Postoperative SICU Admission: 0 vs 0 vs 3 Wound Infection: 2 vs vs 1 vs 8 Blood Transfusion: 3 vs 2 vs 15

Author/ Year	Operations	Number of patients	Operation time (min)	EBL (ml)	Conversion rate	Intraoperative complications	Hospital stay (days)	Postoperative complications
Patzkowsky et al., 2013	RH vs LH	288 vs 257	99.4±166.5 vs 100.9±136.4	231±64.2 vs 228.1±60.1	5 vs 16	Viscus injury: 5 vs 3 Blood transfusion: 1 vs 3	NM	Vesicovaginal fistula: 0 vs 1 Vaginal cuff complications: 14 vs 6 Vaginal cuff dehiscence: 1 vs 5 Thrombotic event: 0 vs 2 Pneumonia: 2 vs 0 Urinary tract infection: 20 vs 7 Urinary retention: 31 vs 11 Ileus: 2 vs 0 Wound complications: 9 vs 5 Reoperation: 5 vs 13
Saceanu et al., 2013	RH vs LH vs AH	29 vs 30 vs 30	183.9±8.91 vs 111.5±4.78 vs 91.55±6.26	199.3±12.8 vs 285.3±12.56 vs 417.7±16.53	0 vs 2	NM	2.39±0.07 vs 3.75±0.43 vs 8.09±0.76	Minor: 4 vs 6 vs 10

Abbreviations: RH = robotic-assisted laparoscopic hysterectomy, LH = laparoscopic hysterectomy, AH = abdominal hysterectomy, LAVH = laparoscopic-assisted vaginal hysterectomy, NM = not mentioned, PE = pulmonary embolism.

Chapter 28

Single Port Hysterectomy

Table. Possible indications and contraindications in the utilization of single site port robotic assisted hysterectomy

Indications	Contraindications
• Low body mass index. • Good physical status of the patient. • Clear surgical history. • Young age.	• Metastatic disease / carcinomatosis. • Poor pulmonary function. • Extensive prior umbilical surgery. • Morbid obesity. • Central obesity. • Uterus of large dimension.

a) Low lithotomy position with the legs at stirrups. The arms are placed at the sides of the patient.
b) After the intubation, a Foley catheter and a uterine manipulator are positioned.
c) A laparoscopic motorized endoscope holder such as ViKY® (Endocontrol Medica, La Tronche, France) can also be positioned so as to be utilized as surgeon's third hand.
d) A vertical incision (up to 30 mm) is made at the inferior part of umbilicus via an open Hasson approach.
e) A single-port multiple channel device (a high-definition camera, two or more assistant ports, insufflator cannulae) is placed through the incision with the use of a Mayo-Guyon clamp. Insufflation of CO_2 (up to 12 mmHg) into the abdominal cavity for the creation of pneumoperitoneum.

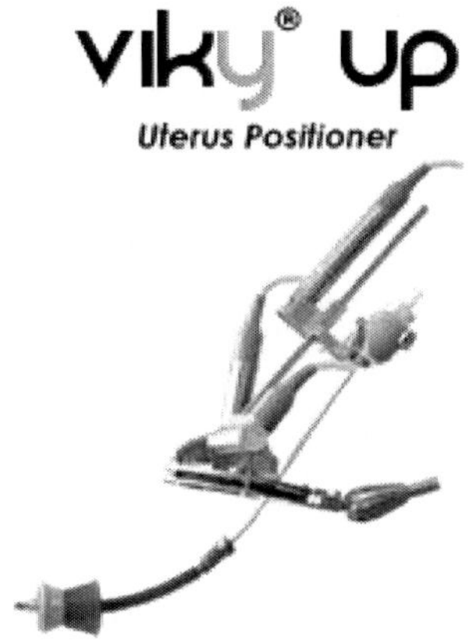

Viky-up.

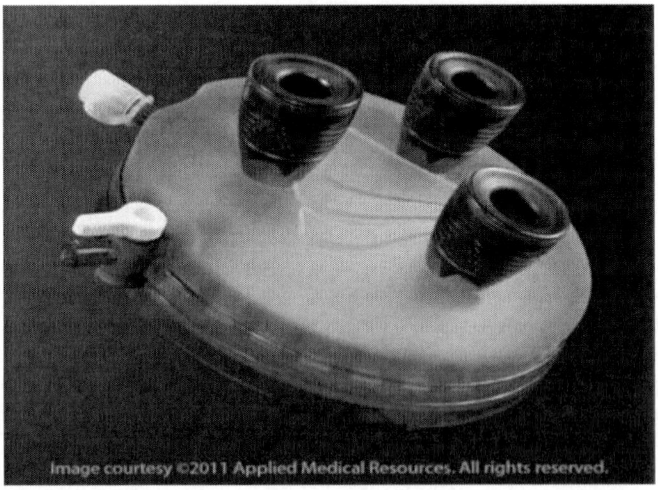

Single-port system.

At present time, there are available several port systems. Some of these single use multichannel single-port systems include the GelPort (Applied Medical, Rancho Santa Margarita, CA), Triport-Quadport (Advanced Surgical Concepts, Wicklow, Ireland), the SILS port system (Covidien, Mansfield, MA), OctoPort (C-308, High Tech Center, Seoul, Korea) and the surgical glove made port.

a) The patient then is placed in a Trendelenburg position (in 30–35º). The da Vinci robot is docked between the legs. The camera is positioned at the upper port access so as to avoid collisions between the other instruments.
b) An endoscopic suction device and a standard atraumatic grasper could be placed through the assistant ports. Pelvis can be exposed by holding back both the small bowel and the rectosigmoid colon with the use of atraumatic laparoscopic graspers.

c) The uterus and the ovaries are inspected. Both the round ligament and the infundibulopelvic ligament are coagulated and ligated. Retroperitoneal space is opened to identify the ureter.
d) Uterine arteries are coagulated and ligated. The bladder is dissected below the level of the colpotomy cup and then a colpotomy is performed.
e) Uterus and adnexae are removed either through the vaginal canal or through port site incision (placed in a plastic bag). The vaginal cuff is sealed with sutures, in preference with barbed ones. The ovaries could be preserved, in younger patients with benign diagnosis.
f) In case it is necessary to proceed to pelvic lymphadenectomy, peritoneum is incised along to the external iliac artery.
g) The external iliac vessels are successively cauterized and moved anterior and laterally in order to avoid any injury to the genitofemoral nerve, which is situated anteriorly along the muscle psoas.
h) With a Cadiere grasper, paravesical and pararectal spaces are created by gentle dissection. Lymph nodes from the mid portion of the common iliac artery superiorly, to the circumflex iliac vein inferiorly and from the mid-portion of the psoas muscles laterally, to the ureters and the hypogastric artery and vein medially are removed.
i) Nodal tissue present in the obturator fossa is also dissected. All the excised lymph nodes are positioned in plastic bags and through an assistant port. In the same mode is performed the dissection of the left pelvic lymph nodes.

Limitations

- instrument crowding
- absence of triangulation
- the use of surgical ports with a larger outer cap, such as the Gel- POINT access device, can increase the instrument distance
- the various movements of the robotic arms can cause gas leaking reducing the necessary pneumoperitoneum, while a query could also be raised regarding the increased possibility of port site metastasis in such patients in the future
- the learning curve of the technique

Chapter 29

Suturing Techniques

- In robotic surgery, the most popular suturing technique is the knotless method.
- Knotless barbed sutures are monofilament absorbable sutures with specially designed cutting barbs which are orientated in an opposite direction to the needle.
- Sutures can have needle in one end or on both ends while the formed barbs change direction at the middle of the suture. The presence of these barbs makes the suture to grab the tissue, without allowing the suture to slide back. The continuous suturing becomes very simple, without the need to tie a knot at the end. Another advantage of barbed sutures is that the tensile strength is distributed equally along the entire length of the wound.
- At the present time, there are three types of knotless barbed commercially available: Quill SRS (Quill Self-Retaining System; Angiotech Pharmaceuticals), which was the first ever utilized bidirectional barbed suture in gynecologic laparoscopy, the V-Loc Absorbable Wound Closure device (Covidien), which has only one needle and a loop at the end for unidirectional technique and the Stratafix (Ethicon). Barbed sutures are available in both absorbable and non-absorbable monofilament materials.

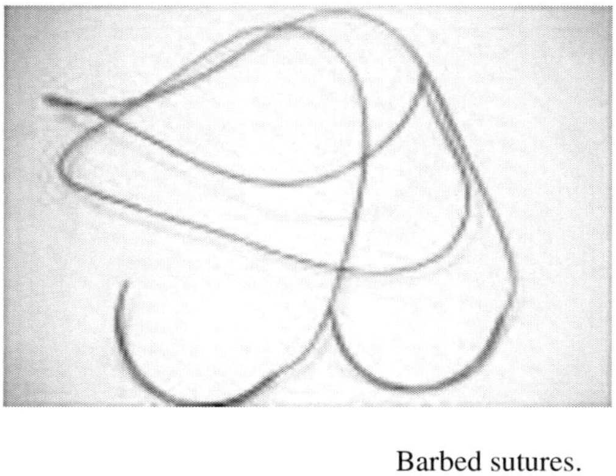

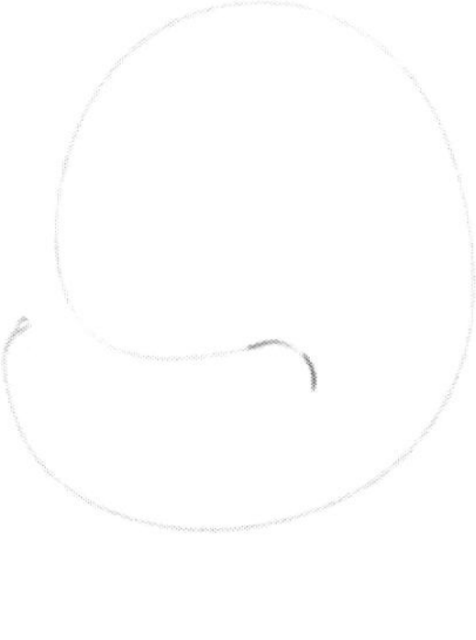

Barbed sutures.

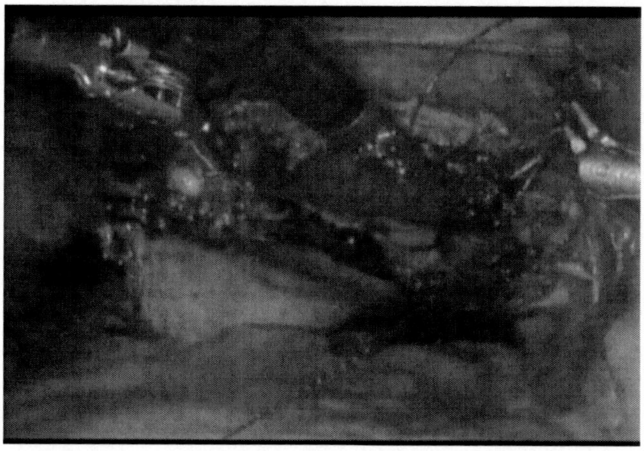

Vaginal vault closure.

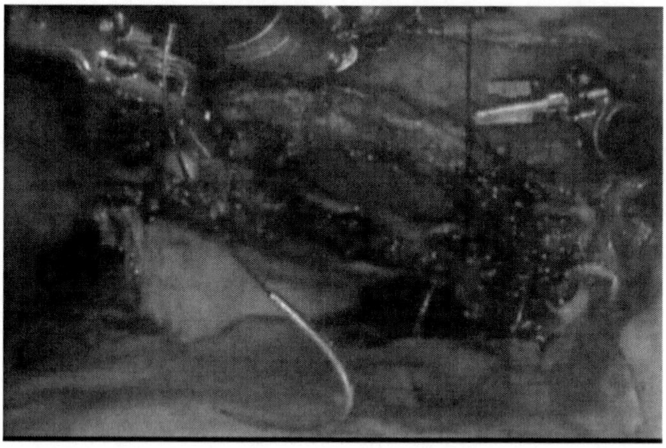

Vaginal vault closure.

- The utilization of barbed suture can decrease the closure time and it can be performed in a more atraumatic mode.
- The learning curve of sewing with barbed suture is minimal compared to traditional suturing.
- The most common problem occurring with the use of barbed sutures is vaginal cuff dehiscence.
- Bowel obstruction has been described which might be attributable to the increased risk of adhesions and inflammation caused by the barbs entrapped in the suture. Events of intestinal obstruction can be avoided if the free edge is cut sufficiently short.
- The application of barbed suture is more expensive compared to conventional ones. The barbed sutures cost three times more than traditional absorbable sutures.

Chapter 30

Robotic Gynaecology in Adolescents

Robot Da Vinci could be used similarly to laparoscopy as the 'gold- standard' diagnostic tool for:

a. Endometriosis

A careful systematic evaluation of the abdomen/pelvis beginning with the pouch of Douglass followed by the ovarian fossae, the uterosacral ligaments. Then the abdomen is evaluated. Typical findings in adolescents would be small clear papules and red lesions.

b. Pelvic Inflammatory Disease

The early diagnosis is the key to reduce the sequelae of this infection.

c. Adnexal Mass

Functional ovarian cysts or haemorrhagic cysts are the most common cystic pelvic masses.Benign mature teratoma (dermoid cyst) is the most frequent neoplasm. Malignant pelvic neoplasms of gynecologic origin are rare in adolescents and include sex cord stromal tumors (granulosa cell, theca cell, Leydig and Sertoli cells) and germ cell tumors (dysgerminoma, malignant teratoma, endodermal sinus tumor, embryonal carcinoma, choriocarcinoma). The sensitivity is 100% for diagnosis of malignancy. The majority of benign ovarian neoplasms could be managed robotically as well as staging in early ovarian malignancies.

Surgical steps of robotic ovarian cystectomy:

- Ovarian capsule incision.
- Dissection of the alveolar tissue between the cyst and the ovarian capsule.
- The cyst is removed from the ovarian capsule and base of the ovary.
- Haemostatic running mattress suture is placed starting at the upper pole where the suture is tied.
- The cyst is removed with the ovary intact.

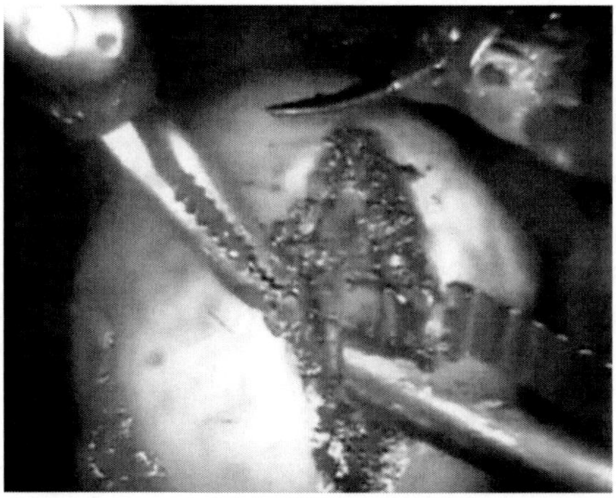

Ovarian capsule incision.

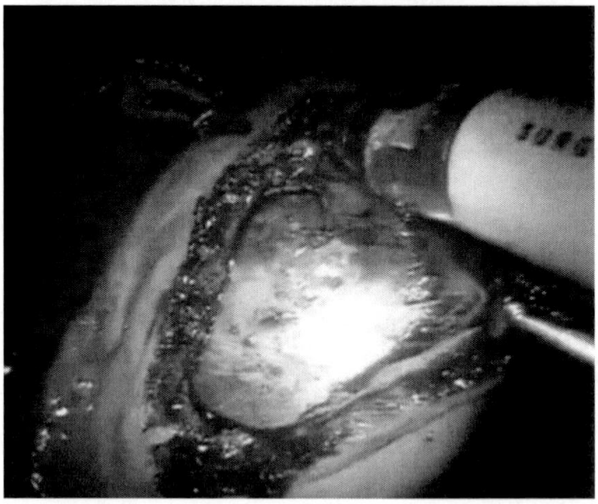

Cyst removal.

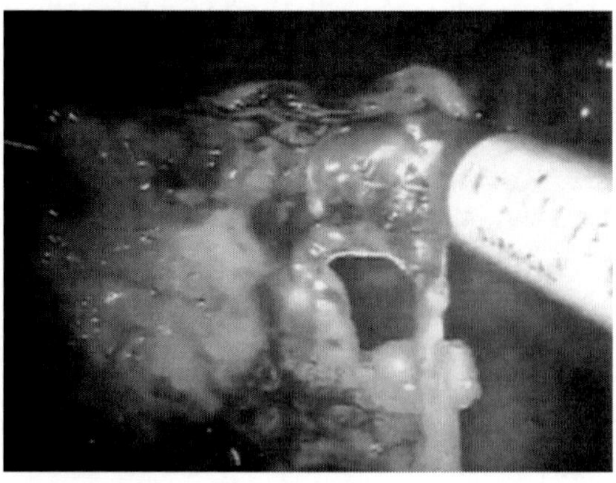

Cyst removal.

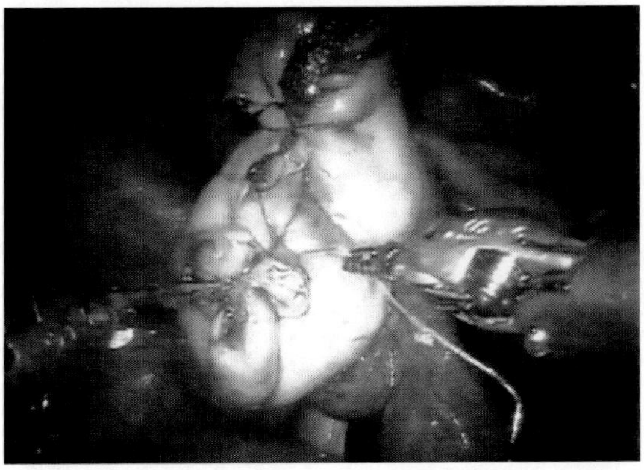

Haemostatic suture.

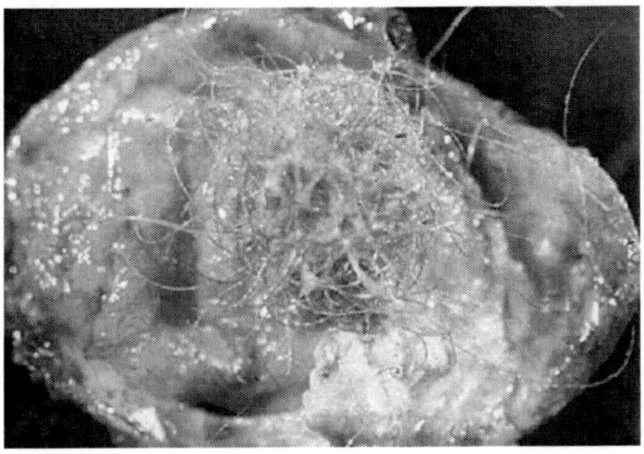

Dermoid cyst.

d. Ovarian Torsion

To improve chances of ovarian salvage or to perform a robotic adnexectomy.

e. Müllerian Malformations

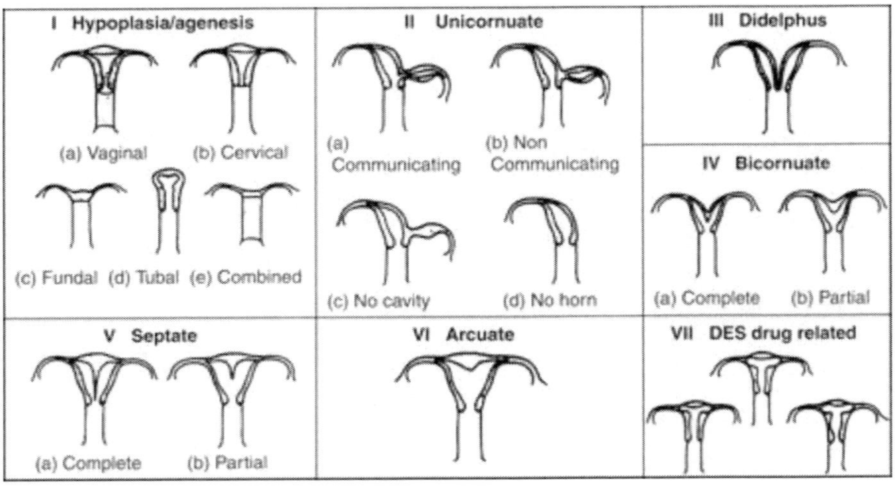

Uterine malformations.

Diagnosis and treatment of obstructed uterovaginal or uterine duplication malformations can be achieved.

Diagnosis of an asymmetric bicornuate uterus with an obstructed uterine horn can be achieved.

Removal of obstructed horn.

Diagnosis of Mayer-Rokitansky-Kuster-Hauser syndrome.

Chapter 31

Pregnancy and Robotic Surgery

Changes in the physiology of pregnant woman:

- increase of blood volume
- increase of cardiac output
- increase of per minute ventilation
- decrease in functional residual capacity of the lungs
- increase of oxygen consumption
- augment at carbon dioxide (CO_2) production

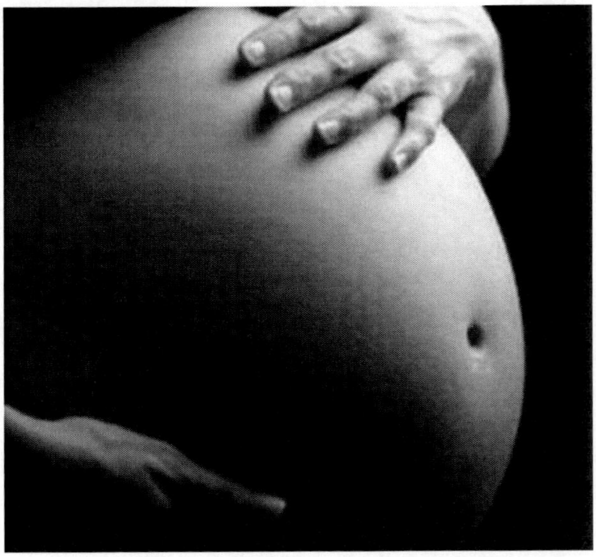

Pregnant.

The pneumoperitoneum in pregnant woman causes hypoxemia and hypercapnia due to:

- reduction of the expansion of diaphragm and of thoracic cavity compliance
- diminution of the functional reserve capacity

With the CO_2 insufflation, at the Trendelenburg position there is increase of the intrathoracic pressure while at the reverse Trendelenburg position there is decrease of the venous return and of the cardiac index.

Regarding fetus:

- Non emergent operations are safer to be performed during the second trimester.
- Emergent operations could be performed during any trimester. The insufflation of CO_2 during the establishment of pneumoperitoneum induces fetal tachycardia and acidosis. The CO2 diffuses in the maternal arterial circulation and is directly correlated to fetal values.

Visualization of the abdomen during robotic surgery becomes difficult due to the size of the uterus, especially in the third trimester. The manipulation of uterus during the operation increases the probability of a preterm labor. In the presence of increased risk of preterm labor, tocolytic medicines should be given for prophylaxis.

Fetal monitoring during robotic surgery in pregnancy is necessary both preoperatively and postoperatively.

For the initial port entry is preferred the open Hassan technique due to the direct visualization of the abdominal cavity. The location of the trocars should be at least 6 cm above the fundus of the uterus.

Carbon dioxide abdominal pressure should be maintained <15mm Hg and if possible <10 mm Hg. The increased intra-abdominal pressure as well as the extra weight of the thick abdominal wall increases airway pressure and decreases ventilatory compliance, having as result the need for higher inspiratory pressure. The application of robotic platform as well as the use of mechanical retractor devices (Laparolift™, Abdo-Lift® LESS) may reduce the required abdominal CO_2 pressure.

Pregnant patients should be placed in a lateral left tilt in order to reduce pressure on the vena cava and sustain a satisfactory venous return, with an optimal tilt of the body at 27 degrees for patients beyond the first trimester of gestation.

Postoperatively, measures should always be taken in order to prevent deep venous thrombosis. The use of sequential compression devices during the operation, compression stockings, prophylactic anticoagulation and the early ambulation are essential for the management of women in pregnancy.

The main advantages of robotic procedures include less manipulation of the gravid uterus, superior visualization, more precise dissection, and fewer conversions to laparotomy. The fundamental advantages of robotic approach, such as the fewer intra and postoperative complications, the lower blood loss and the reduced length of hospital stay pose robotic assisted surgery at a important position among the other minimally invasive surgical techniques for the treatment of pregnant patients.

Chapter 32

Robotic Operations in Obese Patients

Body mass index (BMI) is a simple index which is defined as a person's weight in kilograms divided by the square of his height in meters (kg/m^2).

The WHO suggests that a woman with a BMI greater than or equal to 25 is overweight while with a BMI greater than or equal to 30 is obese.

In 2008, according to the WHO, 35% of adults aged 20 and over were overweight and 11% were obese. More specifically, nearly 300 million women were obese.

Raised BMI is a major risk factor for:

- cardiovascular diseases (mainly heart disease and stroke)
- diabetes mellitus
- hypertension
- obstructive sleep apnea
- osteoarthritis
- cancer (endometrial, breast, and colon).

The risk for endometrial cancer is linked to obesity. More specifically, it is associated with the endocrine and inflammatory effects of fat tissue. Endometrial cancer is most common in postmenopausal women. Unopposed oestrogen plays an important role as a risk factor.

Hysterectomy is the standard of care for endometrial cancer. The procedure is traditionally performed through a laparotomy and has been associated with substantial perioperative morbidity. Minimally invasive options could be used and are associated with lower morbidity and shorter hospital stay. In the last decade, robotic hysterectomy is widely used even for obese or morbidly obese patients. The main advantages include increased dexterity provided by the robotic Arms, high-definition 3-dimensional vision system and retracting capability of the third robotic arm. Moreover, the robotic arms could be used to lift the weight of the abdominal wall ("Italian manoeuver").

Technique

- Anaesthetic review and ITU bed might be necessary depending on the commorbidities
- Preoperative bowel preparation
- The patient is self-positioning in the dorso-lithotomy position
- Bariatric bed is used
- Some teams are using shoulder blocks, but it is suggested to be avoided in order to prevent brachial plexus injury in the event that the patient slides while in the steep Trendelenburg position. Instead, an egg-crate foam mattress is suggested to reduce sliding

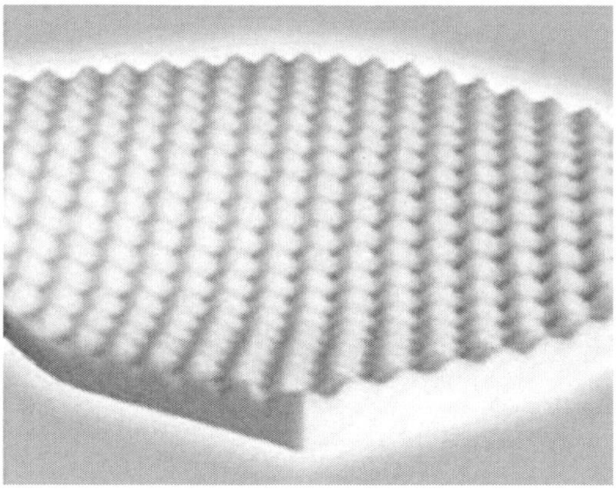

Egg-crate foam mattress.

- Intermittent pneumatic compression boots are used to prevent deep venous thrombosis. The patient is going to have low molecular weight heparin adjusted to her weight for a month.

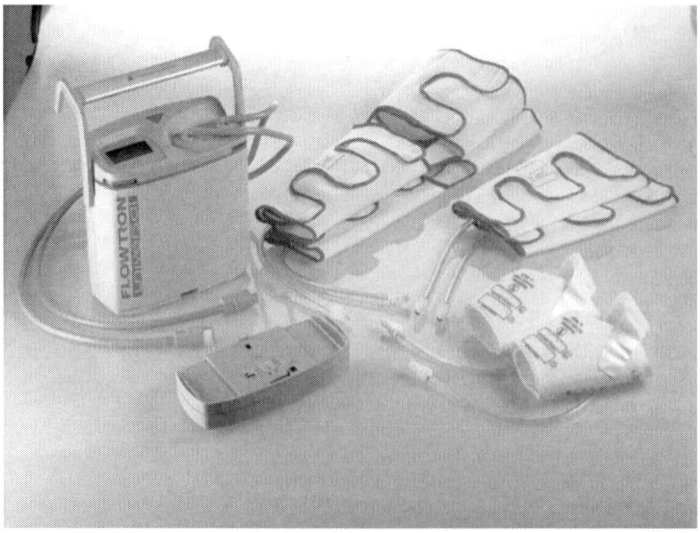

Compression boots.

- After general anaesthesia, the arms are placed in the arms-tucked "military" position.
- One dose of intraoperative cephalosporin
- Uterine manipulator is used (RUMI, V-care)
- The panniculus of the abdomen could be elevated with tapes or towels.
- The pneumoperitoneum is maintained at 15 mm Hg throughout the procedure
- Extra-long laparoscopic trocars might be necessary
- Usually, the camera trocar is inserted several centimeters above the umbilicus
- The other 4 trocars are placed approximately 10 cm lateral in a reverse "W" figure

Anaesthetic concerns:

Pneumoperitoneum and steep Trendelenburg position significantly increase mean arterial pressure (MAP) and systemic vascular resistance (SVR). Trendelenburg position also increases stroke volume while pneumoperitoneum decreases aortic diameter. No significant changes are usually noted in cardiac output or stroke volume.

A recent German study showed that the number of perioperative complications was not different between the patients with normal BMI compared to those with high BMI in women undergoing robotic hysterectomy. However, a significant difference in women's positioning time was found between normal weighted and obese groups (35 and 55 min, $p < 0.001$).

Robotic surgery may offer particular advantages in obese patients with no conversions and no wound complications. Obese patients who undergo robotic surgery have shorter hospital stay, less postoperative pain, and fewer wound complications when compared with obese patients who undergo an open procedure.

Chapter 33

Elderly Patients and Robotic Surgery

The elderly patient is considered a high-risk patient as a result of the presence of a large number of co-morbidities and the absence of functional reserves.

Reduced respiratory vital capacity, decreased renal function, decreased cardiac stroke and blood volume are among the principal alterations present at elderly patients.

In elderly patients, an ASA (American Society of Anesthesiology) score 2 or higher is correlated with increased complications and mortality. Moreover, the age of 70 years old or higher represent an independent factor for prolonged hospital stay and increased risk of in-hospital mortality.

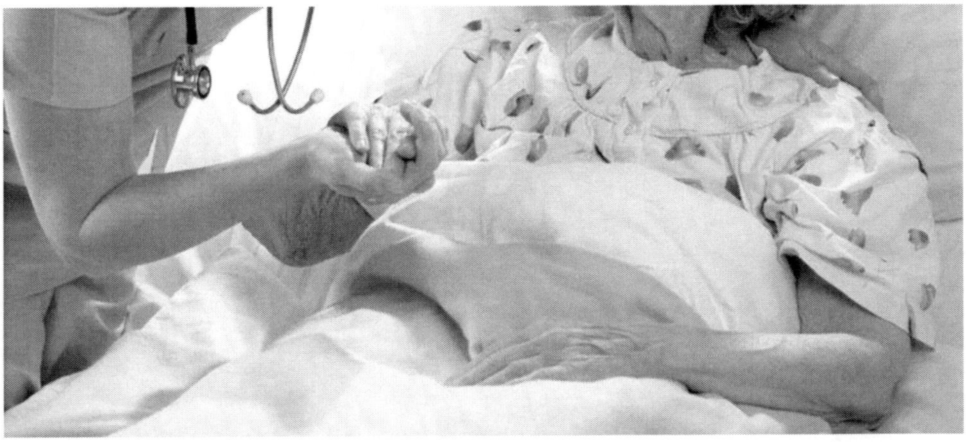

Care of elderly patient.

The establishment of pneumoperitoneum causes further reduction of the functional residual capacity of the lungs and of the respiratory compliance. The insufflation in the abdominal cavity of CO_2 causes hypercapnia and academia as consequence of absorption of CO_2 through the peritoneal membrane. Physiological modifications in ventilation can prevent these alterations; however in patients with underlying pulmonary co-morbidities these changes may be not tolerated.

The loss of blood has an immediate impact on cardiac performance by influencing the preload, the afterload and the myocardial contractility as well. Nevertheless, in elderly patients changes at the cardiac function may be difficult due to the absence of sufficient cardiac reserves.

Minimally invasive surgical techniques, such as the robotic assisted surgery, in combination with enhanced recovery programs may assist at achievement of better surgical outcomes in elderly population. The application of robotic surgery in patients with underlining co-morbidities offers optimal post operative outcomes:

- decreased post operative complications
- fewer wound complications
- minimal rates of conversion to open
- decreased hospital stay
- earlier return to everyday activities

The implementation of organized enhanced recovery programs in order to reduce both the morbidity and postoperative mortality among the elderly population should include elements:

- patient education (direct participation of the patient to her therapy)
- sufficient analgesia
- equilibrate fluid administration
- early mobilization and early feeding

The central aim of enhanced recovery programs is the achievement of reduced hospitalization and single day hospital stay if possible.

Chapter 34

Possile Role of Da Vinci Robot in Uterine Transplantation

Indications:

- history of hysterectomy at a young age for malignant uterine tumors or benign diseases such as fibroids or adenomyosis
- emergency peripartum hysterectomy
- congenital uterine infertility e.g. Mayer-Rokitansky-Kuster-Hauser syndrome

History of uterine transplantation in humans:

- First, human uterine transplantation was attempted in Saudi Arabia in 2002, but necrosis of the graft occurred 99 days after surgery and the attempt failed.
- Second case was a 21-year-old patient with Mayer-Rokitansky-Kuster-Hauser syndrome in Turkey who had normal cycles and an implanted embryo.
- Nine women in Sweden till now have successfully received transplanted uterus.

Anatomy:

The uterine artery originates bilaterally from the anterior division of the hypogastric artery and runs medialward on the levator ani muscle toward the cervix. At the side of the uterus, it ascends between the two layers of the broad ligament to the junction of the salpinx and uterus. Branches of the uterine artery form anastomoses with branches from the ovarian artery in the upper part of the broad ligament.

Uterine veins form plexuses that end into the internal iliac vein. They merge downward with the vaginal plexus and upward with the utero-ovarian plexus, draining into inferior vena cava on the right and in the renal vein on the left.

Technique:

- Hysterectomy of the donor uterus with preserved uterine vessels all the way to internal iliacs plus extended round and uterosacral ligaments
- Preparation of vessels ex vivo
- The vaginal wall of the excised uterus is anastomosed with the vaginal stump, using the prosthetic valve-suturing technique used in cardiac valve replacement.

- Vascular anastomosis (Internal iliac arteries of the donor uterus end-to-end anastomosed with that on the recipient as well as the uterine veins end-to-end anastomosed with internal iliac veins and proximal utero-ovarian veins
- Fixation of ligaments

Advantages:

- Micro-vascular anastomosis techniques easier ?
- three-dimensional (3D) view
- wrist-like motion of the robotic arms
- lower blood loss ?
- fewer wound complications
- ideal for obese patients
- reduced length of hospital stay ?
- faster return to normal activities ?

Disadvantages:

- Decision on how the donor uterus is going to be inserted in the abdominal cavity
- No previous experience
- Ethical concerns of uterine transplantation
- Necessity for extensive evaluation of the recipient and donor by an experienced multidisciplinary transplantation team (major risks related to surgery, immunosuppression, and possible pregnancy)

Chapter 35

Pre- and Postoperative Management of Patients Undergoing Robotic Operations

Preoperatively:

A pre-operative assessment appointment is scheduled with the doctor +/- a nurse practitioner.

The patient is signing the consent form where she is informed about the type of operation and the possible risks of it including: Bleeding, conversion to an open surgery, damage to the bladder, ureters, and to the bowel, blood clots in the legs or lungs, bowel obstruction, hernia, infection, scar tissue, formation of lymphocyst or lymphedema (in cases of lymph node dissection).

Anaesthesiology review might be necessary depending on the general health and comorbidities and it is advised in obese and elderly patients.

Laboratory tests including FBC, U&E, clotting, G&S are requested preoperatively.

Some medications need to be stopped before the surgery such as aspirin and warfarin and converted to low molecular weight heparin.

A smoker is advised to quit 6-8 weeks before surgery, but if she is unable to do so nicotine patch could be suggested.

A bowel preparation is not usually essential for robotic gynaecological operations, but if necessary, the prep is suggested to be completed the night before the operation.

Shower at home before surgery is suggested.

Makeup, nail polish, lotion, deodorant, or antiperspirant on the day of surgery should be avoided.

All body piercings and acrylic nails should be removed.

Postoperatively:

The patient is initially going to the recovery room and monitored for a short time before going to the observation unit.

The patient can usually eat and drink 8 hours postoperatively (started usually on a liquid diet).

Cramps, bloatedness or shoulder pain are common complaints.

Antiemetics and pain killers are prescribed.

The urine catheter stays in until the next morning except for radical hysterectomy cases that the catheter stays in for a week or cases which fail TWOC and need reinsertion of catheter.

Compression stockings on the legs could be used to improve circulation.

The patient restarts the routine medications.

Early mobilisation is advised.

Usually the patient is discharged in the first 24 hours.

A family member or a friend should be available to help with the day-to-day activities for a few days after surgery.

At home, it is advised to call the surgeon in cases of fever (>38°C), vaginal bleeding, severe abdominal pain, heavy vaginal discharge, nausea and vomiting, chest pain or difficulty in breathing, oedema, redness, or pain in your legs, changes in urinary or bowel symptoms

Showers are allowed within 24 hours after surgery.

Climbing stairs is permitted with some assistance the first postoperative days. Lifting is advised to be avoided for 4-6 weeks. Driving should be avoided because of the pain medications used, as well as because the patient has restricted ability to make sudden movements due to discomforts from surgery. Normal physical activity could be started with short walks and gradually increase the distance and length of time. More difficult exercise should be started 4-6 weeks postoperatively. Sexual intercourse is advised to be avoided for 6 weeks postoperatively. Most women recover and are back to most activities in 4-6 weeks.

Usually, the patients are having a postoperative appointment 2-3 weeks after the operation in order to be assessed and informed about the histology results

Chapter 36

Anaesthetising for Robotic Pelvic Surgery

Preoperative preparation includes:

- History and physical examination.
- Blood type and antibody screening.
- Blood test and biochemical analysis.
- ECG, chest X ray, pulmonary evaluation.
- One week prior to surgery, interruption of all ASA and antiplatelet medications.
- Psychological preparation.
- Informed consent on the operation and on the probable benefits and complications.
- Fast at least 12 hours prior to the operation.

Set up of anesthesia

- Multimodal analgesia could be initiated as premedication.
- Standard monitoring.
- Insertion of two iv cannulas with an extra extension (at least one should be a large bore).
- Arterial line.
- Arterial blood pressure monitoring (especially for patients with cardiac or pulmonary disease).
- Collocation of padding for axilla, elbows, back and shoulders is recommended.
- Urinary catheterization.
- One dose of intraoperative antibiotic should be administered.

Anesthesia technique

- Once da Vinci® system is docked, is advised not to change the position of the surgical table.

- During the docking period of the robot to the patient, neuromuscular blockade is absolute requirement.
- Cover of the eyes.
- Administration of H_2 blockers.
- Oro/nasogastric decompression.
- Antiemetic prophylaxis.
- Intubation (ensure that the endotracheal tube is well secured).
- Control mechanical ventilation to properly handle carbon dioxide absorbed through pneumoperitoneum.
- Ventilation (pressure control ventilation (PEEP up to +20 maximum) is recommended, while PEEP with mean 5 cm H_2O is also advisable).
- Variations in the ventilation are recommended to be through changes of the respiratory rate and not of the tidal volume.
- Maintain the patient paralyzed and sedated until da Vinci® system is undocked.
- Conversion of Iso/Sevo to Desflurane for last hour of the operation.
- Consider leak test before extubation or extubating in the ICU.

Postoperative

- Monitoring at recovery area.
- Maintain elevation of the head of bed.
- Blood gas analysis, haemoglobin and haematocrit analysis.
- In case of signs that suggest subcutaneous emphysema or pneumothorax, chest X ray is indicated.
- Postoperative analgesia including: paracetamol 20-40 mg/kg i.v. / celebrex 200-400 mg p.o..
- If required additional narcotic such as morphine 5-15 .im. / meperidine 50-100 i.m.
- Moderate pain or pain that can not pharmaceutically be treated should be evaluated by the anaesthetist and the surgeon.
- Careful perioperative fluid administration to prevent excessive fluid input and to avoid postoperative oliguria (fluid balance).
- ITU bed is not necessary unless there is further commorbidity.

Possible complications

- Nerve injury as a result of the stirrups and the steep Trendelenburg position (brachial plexus).
- CO_2 subcutaneous emphysema depending on the maximum end-tidal CO2 ($\geq$50 mmHg), the number of operative ports, the duration of operative time (>200 min) and the patient's age.
- Subcutaneous emphysema could lead to pneumothorax, pneumomediastinum and pneumopericardium.
- Venous gas embolism.
- Facial, pharyngeal and laryngeal edema due to the steep Trendelenburg position.

- Ocular injuries and optic neuropathies related to anesthesia and to the steep Trendelenburg position in correlation with significant blood loss (in the majority of the cases the blood loss is minimal).
- Cerebral effects of steep Trendelenburg position. Head-down positioning increases cerebral venous pressure (CVP) and obstacles the venous drainage of the head. The increase of CVP leads to perivascular edema. The development of cerebral edema and the increase of intracranial cerebral pressure (ICP) may cause the increase the vascular resistances in the brain, reduction of the cerebral blood flow and potentially lead to ischemic cerebral injury.

Chapter 37

Enhanced Recovery in Robotic Surgery

The realization of a program of enhanced recovery and its implementation in minimally invasive robotic surgery may reduce length of hospital stay, the rate of complications and mortality. The concept of enhanced recovery includes 3 stages:

- the pre-operative optimization (medical and surgical history of the patient, information on organ function)
- the intra-operative care (reduction of surgical stress, adequate anesthesia)
- the post-operative rehabilitation (satisfactory analgesia, perioperative care pathway, including early feeding and intensive early mobilization)

A well organized enhanced recovery program for robotic surgery in gynecology should include elements that could be implemented: patient education, pre-operative carbohydrate drinks, spinal or local analgesia, equilibrate fluid administration, early feeding and intensive early mobilization. The main aim of such a service is to achieve only a single day hospital stay.

The principal characteristics of an enhanced recovery program in minimally invasive surgery:

Pre-operative care

a) Preoperative fasting
b) Preoperative bowel preparation is not essential
c) Single preoperative dose of antibiotics

Intra-operative care

d) Intraoperative mechanical thromboprophylaxis
e) Maintenance of normothermia
f) Avoidance of nasogastric tubes or abdominal drains
g) Minimal blood loss

h) Use of local anesthetics in key holes closure

Post-operative care

i) Regular use of antiemetics and analgesia
j) Education of relatives in pain and wound care
k) Decreased use of regular opioids as pain killers and laxatives
l) Quick complete deambulation
m) Post-operative thromboprophylaxis

Chapter 38

Possible Complications After Robotic Simple/ Radical Hysterectomy

Patients should be consented preoperatively for all the intra- or post-operative complications.

The proximity of the uterus and adnexae to the bladder, ureters, bowels, nerves and vessels could lead to injury of the adjacent organs intraoperatively.

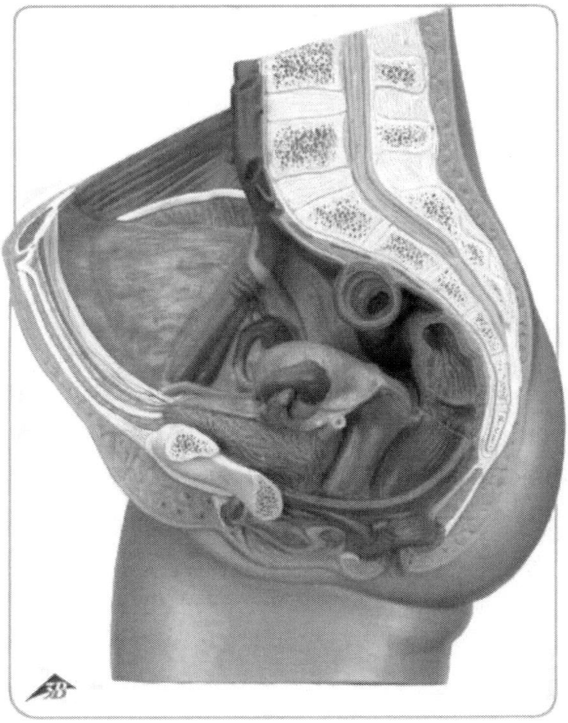

Pelvic anatomy.

Intraoperative complications

a) urinary tract injury (ureteral or bladder injuries): Electrocautery (unipolar or bipolar) is the main reason.

b)

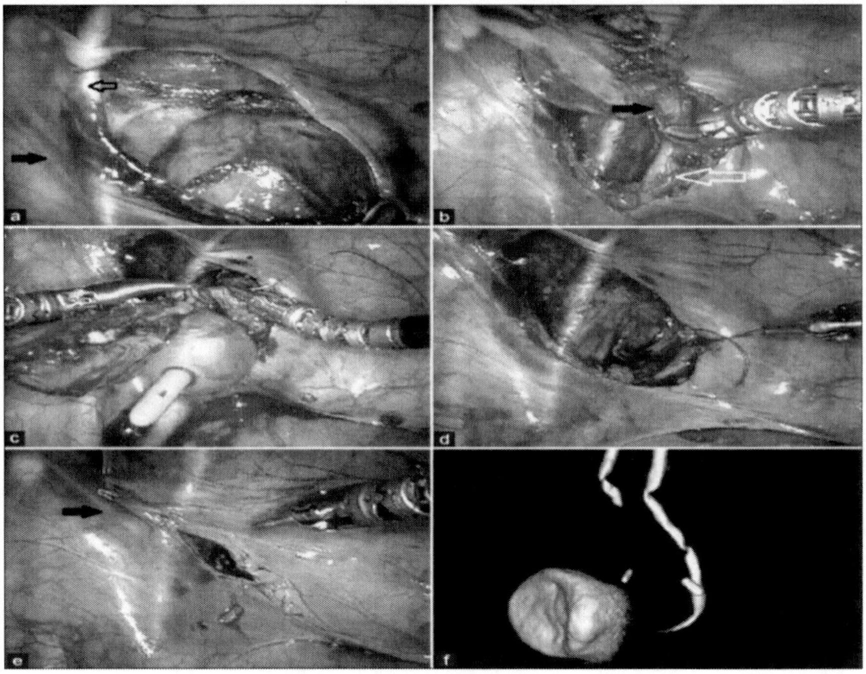

Urinary tract injuries.

c) bowel injury (The mean time from operation to diagnosis is 3 days, but recognition of thermal injury may lag behind 10 days).
d) vessel injury
e) nerve injury
f) abdominal wall vascular injury (inferior epigastric vessel)

Postoperative complications

g) postoperative shoulder pain
h) gas embolism
i) pneumoperitoneum related complications(hypercarbia, subcutaneous emphysema, pneumomediastinum, and pneumothorax)
j) postoperative ileus
k) vaginal cuff dehiscence
l) pelvic abscess
m) deep vein thrombosis

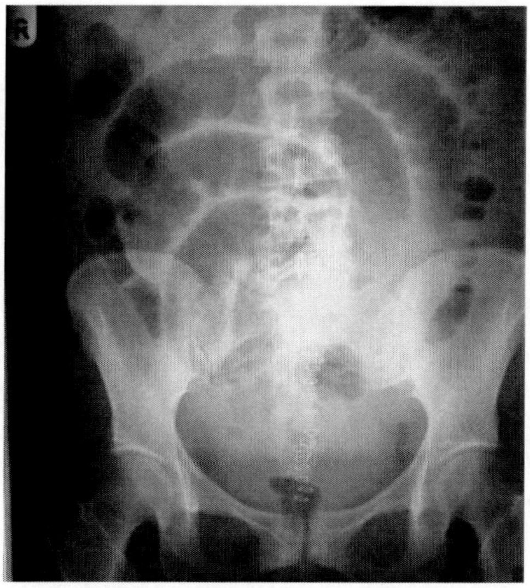

Ileus.

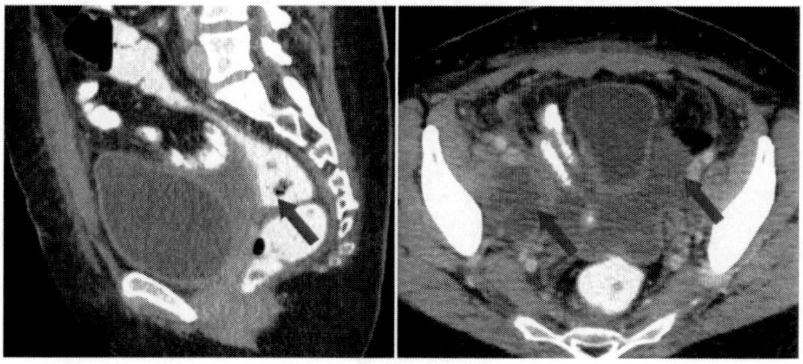

Abscess.

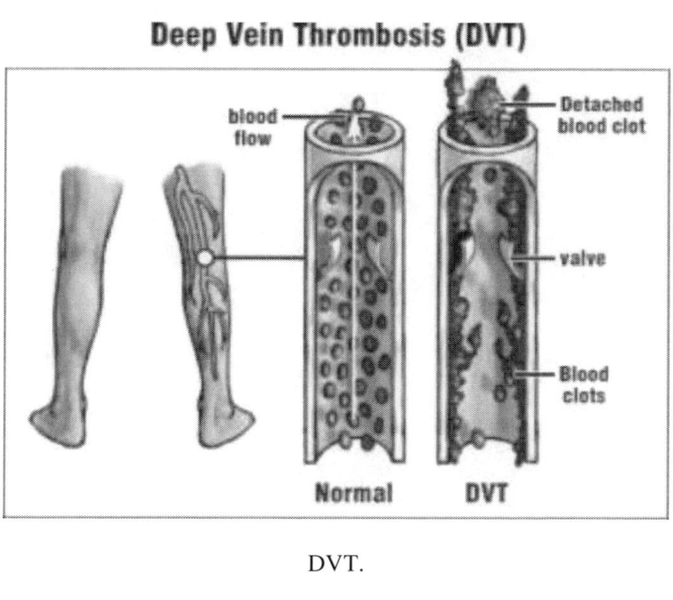

DVT.

n) pulmonary embolism

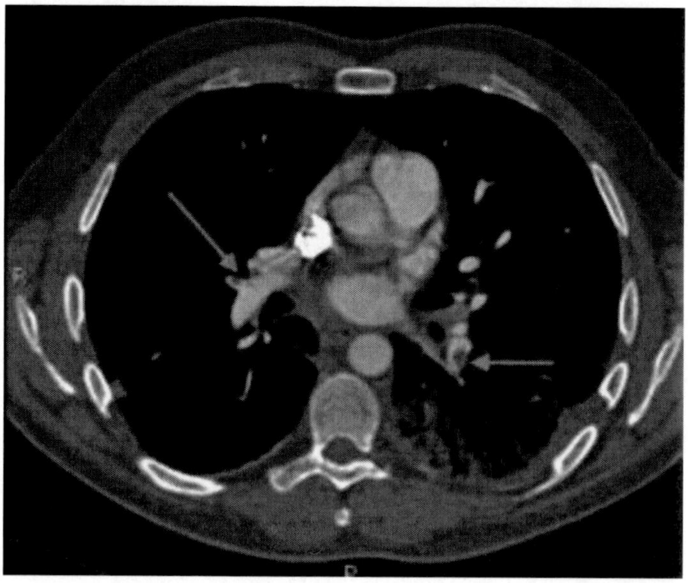

Pulmonary embolism.

o) port-site hernia

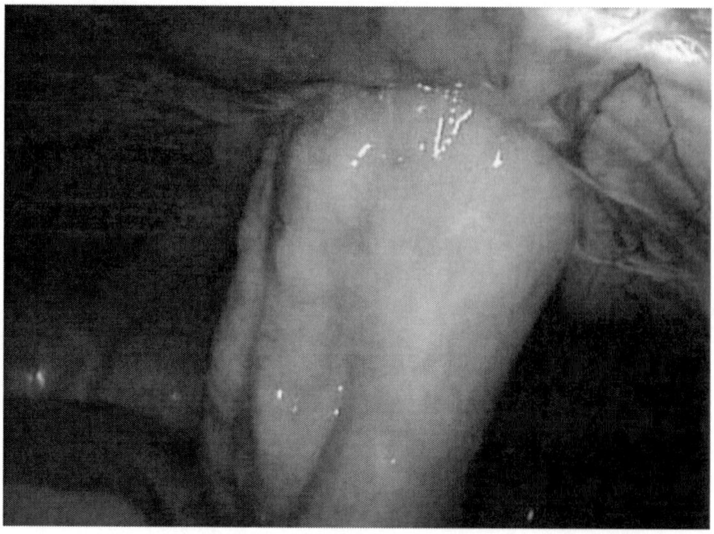

Hernia.

p) UTI
q) pneumonia
r) lymphedema

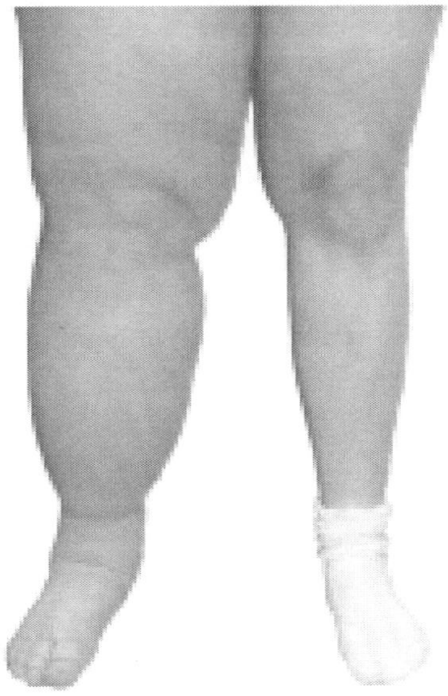

Lymphedema.

a) lymphocele
b) Wound infection
c) Port site metastasis

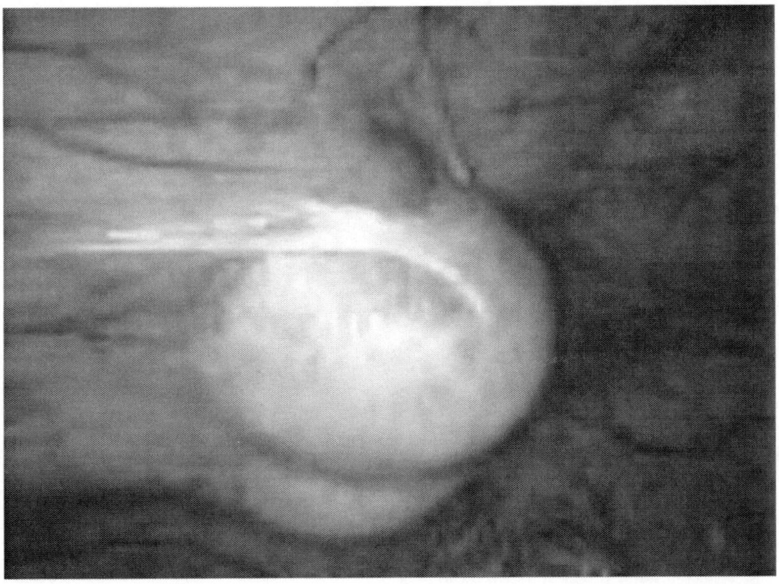

Port site metastasis.

Chapter 39

Port Site Metastases After Robot-Assisted Surgery

- port-site metastasis is defined the development of tumor recurrence at the site of laparoscopic port entrance.
- port-site metastasis is a rare complication, present in <2% of all laparoscopic oncologic operations.
- the etiology of port-site metastases is unknown, probably has a multifactorial origin.
- in robotic surgery, port-site metastasis are identified in the field of gynaecology and urology.

Hypothetic Mechanisms for the Development of Port-Site Metastasis

- patient related

Immunocompetence status, presence of hypoxia and low pH at the wound site can cause angiogenesis and tumor spread at port site.

- tumor related

Biological aggressiveness of the tumor (high grade and stage of the neoplasia)

- wound related

Alterated local and systemic immune response to the pneumoperitoneum

- surgical technique related

– aerolization of the tumor cells into the peritoneal cavity caused by frequent gas insufflation and desufflation
– port site contamination from the repeated introduction of the laparoscopic instruments
– leakage of the utilized gas around the port due to "chimney effect"
– tumor manipulation as consequence of morcellation of the surgical specimen may increase tumor seeding

Management

- Port-site metastasis probably can be avoided by the use of plastic bags or wound protectors to avoid direct contact between the tumour and the wound.
- Surgical excision of the metastatic area is the standard of care.

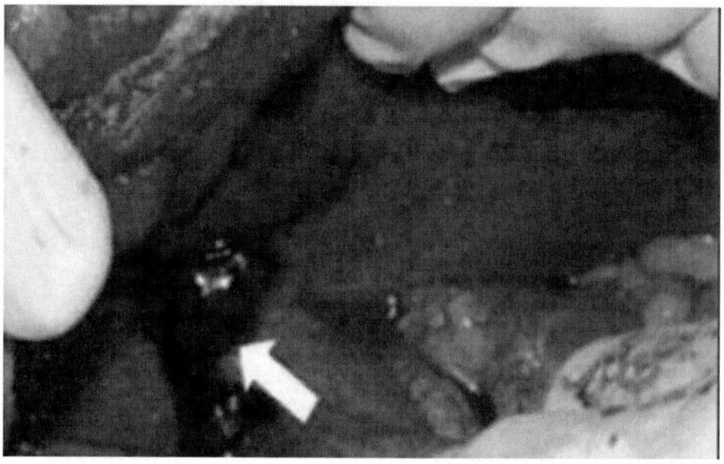

Port site metastasis.

Chapter 40

Ocular Complications and Robotic Surgery

The steep Trendelenburg position is essential for robotic surgery at the pelvic cavity. With the assistance of gravity, abdominal viscera are pulled away from the cavity, permitting to the surgeon to have a free operating field.

The Trendelenburg position represents a not physiological position for the human body that could cause:

- an increase of central venous pressure
- a decrease of cardiac output
- an increase of the blood flow at the direction of the head, resulting in the elevation of the intraocular pressure.

The combination of increased intraocular pressure and the placement of the patient in the Trendelenburg position for period of a few hours or longer may be correlated with the increased risk of developing glaucoma, especially in patients with predisposition to elevated intraocular pressure prior to the operation.

An extremely rare complication correlated to the steep Trendelenburg position in combination with excessive blood loss is the ischemic optic neuropathy. The physiopathology of optic nerve damage probably caused by two different mechanisms: either due to venous infarction as a result of decreased venous outflow or due to the reduced blood supply from the arteries that supply the optic nerve. As preventive measure to both the elevated intraocular pressure and to the ischemic damage of the optic nerve could be the “rest stops”, intervals of reverse Trendelenburg positioning during the operation of robotic surgery.

Ocular injuries could also be present after an operation of robotic surgery. Corneal abrasions or exposure keratopathy and chemosis are the most common complication related to anesthesia. The first could be thought as result of the use of either eye or plastic tape while the second can be caused by erroneous eye touching and conjunctival edema as consequence of increased administration of intravenous fluids. The utilization of eye transparent occlusive dressings, avoiding eye touching and limiting the quantity of intravenous fluids during steep Trendelenburg position are some of the protective eye measures.

Nevertheless, the presence of conjunctival or facial edema when is observed at the end of the operation should alert the anesthetist for the combined presence of laryngeal edema. In order to avoid this complication, the restriction of intravenous fluids and of the period in which patient is positioned with the head-down are crucial.

For the reasons above, some studies suggest the preoperative assessment of the patients to evaluate the presence of glaucoma or ocular hypertension, as well as presence of ischemic events.

Chapter 41

Training in Da Vinci Robot

Robotic gynaecological operations by using the da Vinci Surgical System (Intuitive Surgical Inc., Sunnyvale, CA) still require appropriate training as it is associated with a real learning curve. However, lack of training opportunities and lack of structured training are mentioned.

Three standardized robotic surgery training methods (inanimate, virtual reality and in vivo) are suggested:

a. Inanimate method includes didactic lectures and self-directed online-training modules (http://www.intuitivesurgical.com/training/) regarding the benefits and limitations of robotic technology, review of the various robotic systems and standard equipment available for use, introduction lectures to the patient's cart, surgeon's console and vision cart, presentation of robot setup, trocar placement, docking, instrument exchange, clutching, as well as troubleshooting of common technical problems.

b. Virtual reality

There are four virtual reality robotic surgical simulators currently available: RoSS™, dV-Trainer™, SEP Robot™, and da Vinci(®) Skills Simulator™.

The trainees have dedicated time to practice docking, camera setup and instrument exchange, as well as to practice basic robotic skills (e.g. endowrist and camera manipulation, instrument clutching, object manipulation, needle driving, suturing and knot tying, camera navigation, third arm functionality, cautery, and dissection). For example, it is suggested a programme with 10 repetitions of 4 exercises on the da Vinci Skills Simulator: matchboard, ring and rail, suture sponge, and energy switching.

Robotic Gynaecology Training

Trainee ____________________ Patient Hospital No: ____________________

Supervisor ____________________

Date ____________________

	N/A	Observed as bystander	Observed as assistant	Supervised some help	Supervised no help	Independent
Preparation						
Position of patient	☐	☐	☐	☐	☐	☐
Securing patient from slipping	☐	☐	☐	☐	☐	☐
Cleaning and draping	☐	☐	☐	☐	☐	☐
Vaginal phase						
Application of manipulator	☐	☐	☐	☐	☐	☐
Infiltration of methylene blue	☐	☐	☐	☐	☐	☐
Suturing of cervix	☐	☐	☐	☐	☐	☐
Laparoscopy phase						
Veress	☐	☐	☐	☐	☐	☐
Primary trocar	☐	☐	☐	☐	☐	☐
Positioning of secondary trocars	☐	☐	☐	☐	☐	☐
Insertion of secondary trocars	☐	☐	☐	☐	☐	☐
Adhesiolysis	☐	☐	☐	☐	☐	☐
Bowel mobilisation	☐	☐	☐	☐	☐	☐
Peritoneal washings	☐	☐	☐	☐	☐	☐
Docking phase						
Directing the cart in place	☐	☐	☐	☐	☐	☐
Docking telescope arm	☐	☐	☐	☐	☐	☐
Docking left arm	☐	☐	☐	☐	☐	☐
Docking right arm 1	☐	☐	☐	☐	☐	☐
Docking right arm 2	☐	☐	☐	☐	☐	☐
Deciding choice of instruments	☐	☐	☐	☐	☐	☐
Checking instruments	☐	☐	☐	☐	☐	☐
Parking instruments in place	☐	☐	☐	☐	☐	☐
Lifting the abdominal wall with arm	☐	☐	☐	☐	☐	☐
Choice of energy settings	☐	☐	☐	☐	☐	☐

Console phase

	N/A	Observed as bystander	Observed as assistant	Supervised some help	Supervised no help	Independent
Entry into right pelvic side wall	☐	☐	☐	☐	☐	☐
Retroperitoneal localisation of right ureter	☐	☐	☐	☐	☐	☐
Securing right IP pedicle	☐	☐	☐	☐	☐	☐
Entry into left pelvic side wall	☐	☐	☐	☐	☐	☐
Retroperitoneal localisation of left ureter	☐	☐	☐	☐	☐	☐
Securing left IP pedicle	☐	☐	☐	☐	☐	☐
Uterovesicle peritoneum	☐	☐	☐	☐	☐	☐
Bladder reflection	☐	☐	☐	☐	☐	☐
Right uterine vessels	☐	☐	☐	☐	☐	☐
Right cardinal pedicle	☐	☐	☐	☐	☐	☐
Left uterine vessels	☐	☐	☐	☐	☐	☐
Left cardinal pedicle	☐	☐	☐	☐	☐	☐
Mobilisation of rectouterine space	☐	☐	☐	☐	☐	☐
Entry into vagina	☐	☐	☐	☐	☐	☐
Vaginal cuff creation	☐	☐	☐	☐	☐	☐
Extraction of uterine specimen	☐	☐	☐	☐	☐	☐
Needle driver used	☐	☐	☐	☐	☐	☐
Suturing vaginal vault	☐	☐	☐	☐	☐	☐
Final haemostasis	☐	☐	☐	☐	☐	☐
Infiltration of local anaesthetic	☐	☐	☐	☐	☐	☐

Any other console procedures

Sampling right pelvic lymph nodes	☐	☐	☐	☐	☐	☐
Dissection right pelvic lymph nodes	☐	☐	☐	☐	☐	☐
Bagging right pelvic lymph nodes	☐	☐	☐	☐	☐	☐
Extraction right pelvic lymph nodes	☐	☐	☐	☐	☐	☐
Sampling left pelvic lymph nodes	☐	☐	☐	☐	☐	☐
Dissection left pelvic lymph nodes	☐	☐	☐	☐	☐	☐
Bagging left pelvic lymph nodes	☐	☐	☐	☐	☐	☐
Extraction left pelvic lymph nodes	☐	☐	☐	☐	☐	☐

Finishing

Extracting the instruments	☐	☐	☐	☐	☐	☐
Undocking arms	☐	☐	☐	☐	☐	☐
Removal of trocars	☐	☐	☐	☐	☐	☐
Closure of sheath	☐	☐	☐	☐	☐	☐
Closure of skin	☐	☐	☐	☐	☐	☐

c. In vivo: Standardized robotic surgical tasks in a live porcine model are suggested

It has been shown that after a 4-week robotic training programme the robotic surgical skills of the trainees are improved regardless of specialty, previous robotic experience, and level of training. This could lead to better post-course performance compared to traditional time-based training.

After completing the training programme, the trainee could be assessed after every operation that he/she performs or participate by the following form:

The training should be formally organised in each training centre and should be competence based, instead of time based. Double console systems seem to be a promising tool in surgical education, improving both training and participation in operation lists. A shorter adaption to robotics could be expected in teams with previous experience with standard laparoscopy, however, a stepwise start with simpler cases is the key to achieve a safe adaption to robotic surgery. The learning curve analysis has shown a decrease in docking time and operating time after 10 cases. Proficiency for robotic hysterectomy plus/minus pelvic-paraaortic lymph node dissection for endometrial cancer can be achieved after 20 cases.

Chapter 42

Robotic Patient Form

We suggest the abovementioned form for the patients' management which could be used for their follow-up as well as for research reasons.

Name of the patient:	Name of the Surgeon:	
Hospital number:	Name of the Assistant:	
D.O.B.:		
Height:		
Weight:		
BMI:		
Commorbidities:		
Indication:		
Time in anaesthetic room:	Type of docking:	Side or not
Time in theatre:	Any need for redocking:	Yes/No
Time of patient positioning:	Cytology:	Yes/No
Time that uterine manipulator was inserted:	Total blood loss:	
Time of ports and trocar placement:	Uterine weight:	
Time of docking:	Number of lymph nodes:	
Time started at console:		
Time ended at console:	Any intraoperative complications:	
End of operation:	Any postoperative complications:	
	Hospital stay:	
	Final histology:	
	MDT decision:	Surgical follow-up Chemotherapy Radiotherapy

Chapter 43

Cost Assessment of Robotics in Gynecological Surgery

- one of the principal drawbacks at the dissemination of robotic assisted surgery is the elevated cost of acquisition as well as of maintenance of the robotic platform.
- the only commercially available robotic system is the da Vinci™ surgical system (Intuitive Surgical, CA).
- the costs of the robotic equipment are relatively high, even though these also include the acquisition, training and equipment costs.
- the acquisition cost is over 1 million Euros while the maintenance costs per year are approximately 150,000 Euros.
- it is estimated that the initial capital for the acquisition of robotic platform can be amortized in a period longer of 7 years, which corresponds over 1,000 Euros per patient (under the condition that it is utilized for at least 300 operations / year)
- robotic instruments have a limited number of uses (almost 10 uses per instrument) where the cost per instrument is about over 1,500 Euros.
- even though cost studies are not easy to be carried out, in order for the health care institutions to amortize the costs of robotic technology, an elevated number of patients being operated could be the answer.
- reduction of the operating time is also an important factor that may influence the total surgical costs of the robotic surgery. The operative time is in close relation to the experience of both the operator and the surgical team.
- limited hospital stay in comparison with the open methods can compensate the increased operative expenses of the robotic technique.
- it is essential the creation of specialized robotic units operating on large number of patients per year, the permission of multi-use of the robot by multi-specialties and the minimization of the number of instruments utilized per operationhaving as main aim the cost reduction.

References

Akl MN, Magrina JF, Kho RM, Magtibay PM. Robotic appendectomy in gynaecological surgery: technique and pathological findings. *Int J MedRobot.* 2008 Sep;4(3):210-3.

Alazzam M, Gillespie A, Hewitt M. Robotic surgery in the management of cervical carcinoma. *Arch Gynecol Obstet.* 2011 Oct;284(4):937-43.

Al-Badawi IA, Al-Aker M, Tulandi T. Robotic-assisted salpingostomy for ectopic pregnancy. *J Obstet Gynaecol Can.* 2010 Jul;32(7):627-8.

Almeida OD Jr. Robotic hysterectomy strategies in the morbidly obese patient. JSLS. 2013 Jul-Sep;17(3):418-22.

ASTEC/EN.5 Study Group, Blake P, Swart AM, Orton J, et al. Adjuvant external beam radiotherapy in the treatment of endometrial cancer (MRC ASTEC and NCIC CTG EN.5 randomised trials): pooled trial results, systematic review, and meta-analysis. *Lancet* 2009;373:137-146.

Awad H, Walker CM, Shaikh M, Dimitrova GT, Abaza R, O'Hara J. Anesthetic considerations for robotic prostatectomy: a review of the literature. *J Clin Anesth.* 2012 Sep;24(6):494-504.

Banerjee K, Zafirova Z, Tung A. Corneal abrasions during laparoscopic prostatectomy: mechanisms and prevention. *Anesthesiology* 2008;109:A761.

Bassi A, Tulandi T. Evaluation of total laparoscopic hysterectomy with and without the use of barbed suture. *J Obstet Gynaecol Can.* 2013 Aug;35(8):718-22.

Bedaiwy MA, Barakat EM, Falcone T. Robotic tubal anastomosis: technical aspects. JSLS. 2011 Jan-Mar;15(1):10-5.

Bell A, Relph S, Sivashanmugarajan V, Yoong W. Enhanced recovery programmes: do these have a role in gynaecology? *J Obstet Gynaecol.* 2013 Aug; 33:539-41.

Bernardi LA, Pavone ME. Endometriosis: an update on management. *Womens Health* (Lond Engl). 2013 May;9(3):233-50.

Blazeby JM, Soulsby M, Winstone K, King PM, Bulley S, Kennedy RH. A qualitative evaluation of patients' experiences of an enhanced recovery programme for colorectal cancer. *Colorectal Dis.* 2010 Oct; 12: 236-42

Bodnera J, Augustina F, Wykypiela H, Fisha J, Muehlmanna G, Wetscherb G, Schmida T. The da Vinci robotic system for general surgical applications: a critical interim appraisal. *Swiss Med Wkly* 135:674–678, 2005.

Boggess JF, Gehrig PA, Cantrell L, Shafer A, Ridgway M, Skinner EN, et al. A comparative study of 3 surgical methods for hysterectomy with staging for endometrial cancer: robotic assistance, laparoscopy, laparotomy. *Am JObstet Gynecol.* 2008;199:360.e1–360.e9.

Borahay MA, Patel PR, Walsh TM, Tarnal V, Koutrouvelis A, Vizzeri G, Jennings K, Jerig S, Kilic GS. Intraocular pressure and steep Trendelenburg during minimally invasive gynecologic surgery: is there a risk? *J Minim Invasive Gynecol.* 2013 Nov-Dec;20(6):819-24.

Boustead GB, Feneley MR. Pelvic exenterative surgery for palliation of malignant disease in the robotic era. *Clin Oncol* (R Coll Radiol) 2010;22:740-6.

Brill AI, Cohen BM. Fundamentals of peritoneal access. *J Am Assoc Gynecol* Laparosc. 2003;10:286–297.

Bulletti C, Montini A, Setti PL, Palagiano A, Ubaldi F, Borini A. Vaginal parturition decreases recurrence of endometriosis. 5. *Fertil Steril.* 2010 Aug;94(3):850-5.

Bulun SE. Uterine fibroids. *N Engl J Med.* 2013 Oct 3;369(14):1344-55.

Caillet M, Vandromme J, Rozenberg S, Paesmans M, Germay O, Degueldre M. Robotically assisted laparoscopic microsurgical tubal reanastomosis: a retrospective study. *Fertil Steril.* 2010 Oct;94(5):1844-7.

Cardenas-Goicoechea J, Soto E, Chuang L, Gretz H, Randall TC. Integration of robotics into two established programs of minimally invasive surgery for endometrial cancer appears to decrease surgical complications. *J Gynecol Oncol.* 2013 Jan;24(1):21-8.

Carli F, Brown R, Kennepohl S. Prehabilitation to enhance postoperative recovery for an octogenarian following robotic-assisted hysterectomy with endometrial cancer. *Can J Anaesth.* 2012 Aug; 59:779-84.

Carter S, Depasquale S, Stallings S. Robotic-Assisted Laparoscopic Ovarian Cystectomy during Pregnancy. *AJP Rep.* 2011 Sep;1(1):21-4.

Carvalho L, Abrão MS, Deshpande A, Falcone T. Robotics as a new surgical minimally invasive approach to treatment of endometriosis: a systematic review. *Int J Med Robot.* 2012 Jun;8(2):160-5.

Chandler JG, Corson SL, Way LW. Three spectra of laparoscopic entry access injuries. *J Am Coll Surg.* 2001;192:478–91

Chen CC, Falcone T. Robotic gynecologic surgery: past, present, and future. *Clin Obstet Gynecol.* 2009 Sep;52(3):335-43.

Connolly M, Seligman J, Kastenmeier A, Goldblatt M, Gould JC. Validation of a virtual reality-based robotic surgical skills curriculum. *Surg Endosc.* 2014 Jan 1.

Curet MJ. Port site metastases. *Am J Surg.* 2004 Jun;187(6):705-12.

Davis MA, Adams S, Eun D, Lee D, Randall TC. Robotic-assisted laparoscopic exenteration in recurrent cervical cancer Robotics improved the surgical experience for 2 women with recurrent cervical cancer. *Am JObstet Gynecol* 2010;202:663 e1.

Dharia Patel SP, Steinkampf MP, Whitten SJ, Malizia BA. Robotic tubal anastomosis: surgical technique and cost effectiveness. *Fertil Steril.* 2008 Oct;90(4):1175-9.

Donnellan NM, Mansuria SM. Small bowel obstruction resulting from laparoscopic vaginal cuff closure with a barbed suture. *J Minim InvasiveGynecol* 2011;18:528-30.

Einarsson JI, Chavan NR, Suzuki Y, Jonsdottir G, Vellinga TT, Greenberg JA. Use of bidirectional barbed suture in laparoscopic myomectomy: evaluation of perioperative outcomes, safety, and efficacy. J Minim Invasive Gynecol 2011;18:92-5.

Escobar PF, Haber GP, Kaouk J, Kroh M, Chalikonda S, Falcone T. Single-port surgery: laboratory experience with the da Vinci single-site platform. *JSLS* 2011; 15:136–141.

Escobar PF, Starks D, Fader AN, Catenacci M, Falcone T. Laparoendoscopic single-site and natural orifice surgery in gynecology. *Fertil Steril* 2010; 94:2497–2502.

Fageeh W, Raffa H, Jabbad H et al. Transplantation of the human uterus. *Int JGynecol Obstet* 2002; 7:245–251.

Falabella A, Moore-Jeffries E, Sullivan MJ, Nelson R, Lew M. Cardiac function during steep Trendelenburg position and CO2 pneumoperitoneum for robotic-assisted prostatectomy: a trans-oesophageal Doppler probe study. *Int J Med Robot.* 2007 Dec;3(4):312-5.

Fanfani F, Gagliardi ML, Zannoni GF, et al. Total laparoscopic hysterectomy in early-stage endometrial cancer using an intrauterine manipulator: is it a bias for frozen section analysis? Case-control study. *J Minim InvasiveGynecol* 2011;18:184-8.

Fechner AJ, Alvarez M, Smith DH, Al-Khan A. Robotic-assisted laparoscopic cerclage in a pregnant patient. *Am J Obstet Gynecol.* 2009 Feb;200(2):e10-1.

Foell K, Finelli A, Yasufuku K, Bernardini MQ, Waddell TK, Pace KT, Honey RJ, Lee JY. Robotic surgery basic skills training: Evaluation of a pilot multidisciplinary simulation-based curriculum. *Can Urol Assoc J.* 2013 Nov;7(11-12):430-4.

Foshager MC, Walsh JW. CT anatomy of the female pelvis: a second look. *Radiographics.* 1994 Jan;14(1):51-64.

Francis P. Evolution of robotics in surgery and implementing a perioperative robotics nurse specialist role. *AORN J.* 2006 Mar;83(3):630-42, 644-6, 649-50

Francis P1, Winfield HN. Medical robotics: the impact on perioperative nursing practice. *Urol Nurs.* 2006 Apr;26(2):99-104, 107-8.

Frey MK, Ihnow SB, Worley MJ Jr, Heyman KP, Kessler R, Slomovitz BM, Holcomb KM. Minimally invasive staging of endometrial cancer is feasible and safe in elderly women. *J Minim Invasive Gynecol.* 2011 Mar-Apr;18(2):200-4.

Fujii S. Anatomic identification of nerve-sparing radical hysterectomy: a step-by-step procedure. *Gynecol Oncol.* 2008 Nov;111(2 Suppl):S33-41.

Gainsburg DM. Anesthetic concerns for robotic-assisted laparoscopic radical prostatectomy. *Minerva Anestesiol.* 2012 May;78(5):596-604.

Gargiulo AR, Nezhat C. Robot-assisted laparoscopy, natural orifice transluminal endoscopy, and single-site laparoscopy in reproductive surgery. *Semin Reprod Med* 2011; 29:155–168.

Geetha P, Nair MK. Laparoscopic, robotic and open method of radical hysterectomy for cervical cancer: a systematic review. *J Minim AccessSurg* 2012; 8:67–73.

Geppert B, Lönnerfors C, Persson J. Robot-assisted laparoscopic hysterectomy in obese and morbidly obese women: surgical technique and comparison with open surgery. *Acta Obstet Gynecol Scand.* 2011 Nov;90(11):1210-7.

Ghezzi F, Cromi A, Uccella S, Bogani G, Sturla D, Serati M, Bolis P. Nerve-sparing minilaparoscopic versus conventional laparoscopic radical hysterectomy plus systematic. *Surg Innov.* 2013 Oct;20(5):493-501.

Giep BN, Giep HN, Hubert HB. Comparison of minimally invasive surgical approaches for hysterectomy at a community hospital: robotic-assisted laparoscopic hysterectomy, laparoscopic-assisted vaginal hysterectomy and laparoscopic supracervical hysterectomy. *J Robot Surg.* 2010 Sep;4(3):167-175.

Gray's Anatomy: The Anatomical Basis of Clinical Practice, New York: *Churchill Livingstone*, 40th Edition, 2008; 1279-1304.

Hansen A. Swedish surgeons report world's first uterus transplantations from mother to daughter. *BMJ.* 2012 Sep 20;345:e6357.

Hemmerling TM, Terrasini N. Robotic anesthesia: not the realm of science fiction any more. *Curr Opin Anaesthesiol.* 2012 Dec;25(6):736-42.

Highshaw RA, Vakar-Lopez F, Jonasch E, Yasko AW, Matin SF. Port-site metastasis: the influence of biology. *Eur Urol.* 2005 Mar;47(3):357-60.

Holloway RW, Ahmad S. Robotic-assisted surgery in the management of endometrial cancer. *J Obstet Gynaecol Res.* 2012 Jan;38(1):1-8.

Holloway RW, Bravo RA, Rakowski JA, James JA, Jeppson CN, Ingersoll SB, Ahmad S. Detection of sentinel lymph nodes in patients with endometrial cancer undergoing robotic-assisted staging: a comparison of colorimetric and fluorescence imaging. *Gynecol Oncol.* 2012 Jul;126(1):25-9.

Holloway RW, Patel SD, Ahmad S. Robotic surgery in gynecology. *Scand JSurg.* 2009;98(2):96-109.

Holtz DO, Miroshnichenko G, Finnegan MO, Chernick M, Dunton CJ. Endometrial cancer surgery costs: robot vs laparoscopy. *J Minim InvasiveGynecol* 2010;17:500-3.

Hoogendam JP, Hobbelink MG, Veldhuis WB, Verheijen RH, van Diest PJ, Zweemer RP. Preoperative sentinel node mapping with (99m)Tc-nanocolloid SPECT-CT significantly reduces the intraoperative sentinel node retrieval time in robot assisted laparoscopic cervical cancer surgery. *Gynecol Oncol.* 2013 May;129(2):389-94.

Hulka JF. Major vessel injury during laparoscopy. *Am J Obstet Gynecol* 1980; 138:590.

Hurd WW, Wang L, Schmmel MT. A comparison of the relative risk of vessel injury with conical versus pyramidal laparoscopic trocars in a rabbit model. *Am J Obstet Gynecol* 1995; 173: 1731-3.

Iavazzo C, Gkegkes ID. Port site metastases after robot-assisted surgery: a systematic review. *Int J Med Robot.* 2013 Dec;9(4):423-7.

Iavazzo C, Gkegkes ID. Robotic technology for pelvic exenteration in cases of cervical cancer. *Int J Gynaecol Obstet.* 2014 Apr;125(1):15-17.

Iavazzo C, Gkegkes ID. Single-site port robotic-assisted hysterectomy: a systematic review. *Arch Gynecol Obstet.* 2014; 4, 725-731.

Iavazzo C, Gkegkes ID. The role of uterine manipulators in endometrial cancer recurrence after laparoscopic or robotic procedures. *Arch GynecolObstet.* 2013; 5:1003-9.

Iavazzo C, Vorgias G, Akrivos T. Laparoscopic pelvic exenteration: a new option in the surgical treatment of locally advanced and recurrent cervical carcinoma. *Bratisl Lek Listy* 2008;109:467-9.

Jacobi CA, Wenger FA, Ordemann J, Gutt C, Sabat R, Müller JM. Experimental study of the effect of intra-abdominal pressure during laparoscopy on tumour growth and port site metastasis. *Br J Surg.* 1998 Oct;85(10):1419-22.

Jonsdottir GM, Jorgensen S, Cohen SL, et al. Increasing minimally invasive hysterectomy: effect on cost and complications. *Obstet Gynecol.* 2011;117:1142–1149.

Kannisto P, Harter P, Heitz F, Traut A, du Bois A, Kurzeder C. Implementation of robot-assisted gynecologic surgery for patients with low and high BMI in a German gynecological cancer center. *Arch Gynecol Obstet.* 2014 Feb 15.

Kaye AD, Vadivelu N, Ahuja N, Mitra S, Silasi D, Urman RD. Anesthetic Considerations in Robotic-Assisted Gynecologic Surgery. *Ochsner J.* 2013 Winter;13(4):517-524.

Kilic GS, Moore G, Elbatanony A, Radecki C, Phelps JY, Borahay MA. Comparison of Perioperative Outcomes of Total Laparoscopic and Robotically Assisted Hysterectomy for Benign Pathology during Introduction of a Robotic Program. *Obstet Gynecol Int.* 2011;2011:683-703.

Kim ML, Seong SJ. Clinical applications of levonorgestrel-releasing intrauterine system to gynecologic diseases. *Obstet Gynecol Sci.* 2013 Mar;56(2):67-75.

Kizer NT, Powell MA. Surgery in the pregnant patient. *Clin Obstet Gynecol.* 2011 Dec;54(4):633-41.

Krill LS, Bristow RE. Robotic surgery: gynecologic oncology. *Cancer J.* 2013 Mar-Apr;19(2):167-76.

Krishnakumar S, Tambe P, Entry Complications in Laparoscopic Surgery, *J Gynecol Endosc Surg.* 2009 Jan-Jun; 1(1): 4–11

Lambaudie E, Narducci F, Leblanc E, Bannier M, Houvenaeghel G. Robotically-assisted laparoscopic anterior pelvic exenteration for recurrent cervical cancer: report of three first cases. *Gynecol Oncol* 2010;116:582-3.

Lee M, Kim YT, Kim SW, Kim S, Kim JH, Nam EJ. Effects of uterine manipulation on surgical outcomes in laparoscopic management of endometrial cancer: a prospective randomized clinical trial. *Int J GynecolCancer* 2013;23:372-9.

Lee SJ, Calderon B, Gardner GJ, Mays A, Nolan S, Sonoda Y, Barakat RR, Leitao MM Jr. The Feasibility and Safety of Same-Day Discharge after Robotic-Assisted Hysterectomy Alone or with Other Procedures for Benign and Malignant Indications. *Gynecol Oncol.* 2014 Apr 12. pii: S0090-8258(14)00863-4.

Levinson KL, Mahdi H, Escobar PF. Feasibility and optimal dosage of indocyanine green fluorescence for sentinel lymph node detection using robotic single-site instrumentation: preclinical study. *J Minim InvasiveGynecol.* 2013 Sep-Oct;20(5):691-6.

Lim PC. Robotic assisted total pelvic exenteration: a case report. Gynecol Oncol 2009;115:310-1.

Liu H, Lu D, Wang L, Shi G, Song H, Clarke J. Robotic conventional laparoscopic surgery for benign gynaecological disease. *Cochrane Database Syst Rev.* 2012;(2):CD008978.

Liu H, Lu D, Wang L, Shi G, Song H, Clarke J. Robotic surgery for benign gynaecological disease. *Cochrane Database Syst Rev.* 2012 Feb 15;2:CD008978.

Loffer FD, Pent D. Laparoscopy in the obese patient. *Am J Obstet Gynecol* 1976; 125: 104-7

Lopera J, Suri R, Kroma GM, Garza-Berlanga A, Thomas J. Role of interventional procedures in obstetrics/gynecology. *Radiol Clin NorthAm.* 2013 Nov;51(6):1049-66.

Lotan Y. Is robotic surgery cost-effective: no. *Curr Opin Urol* 2012;22:66-9.

Lowery WJ, Leath CA 3rd, Robinson RD. Robotic surgery applications in the management of gynecologic malignancies. *J Surg Oncol.* 2012 Apr 1;105(5):481-7.

Lv D, Wang X, Shi G.. Perioperative enhanced recovery programmes for gynaecological cancer patients. *Cochrane Database Syst Rev.* 2010 Jun; 16:CD008239.

Magrina JF, Magtibay PM. Robotic nerve-sparing radical parametrectomy: feasibility and technique. *Int J Med Robot.* 2012 Jun;8(2):206-9.

Magrina JF, Zanagnolo V, Giles D, Noble BN, Kho RM, Magtibay PM. Robotic surgery for endometrial cancer: comparison of perioperative outcomes and recurrence with laparoscopy, vaginal/laparoscopy and laparotomy. *Eur J Gynaecol Oncol* 2011;32:476-80.

Manceau G1, Karoui M, Werner A, Mortensen NJ, Hannoun L. Comparative outcomes of rectal cancer surgery between elderly and non-elderly patients: a systematic review. *Lancet Oncol.* 2012 Dec;13(12):e525-36.

Marano A, Priora F, Lenti LM, Ravazzoni F, Quarati R, Spinoglio G. Application of fluorescence in robotic general surgery: review of the literature and state of the art. *World J Surg.* 2013 Dec;37(12):2800-11.

Marnitz S, Kohler C, Muller M, Behrens K, Hasenbein K, Schneider A. Indications for primary and secondary exenterations in patients with cervical cancer. *Gynecol Oncol* 2006;103:1023-30.

Martin S. The role of the first assistant in robotic assisted surgery. *Br JPerioper Nurs.* 2004 Apr;14(4):159-63.

Matthews CA, Reid N, Ramakrishnan V, Hull K, Cohen S. Evaluation of the introduction of robotic technology on route of hysterectomy and complications in the first year of use. *Am J Obstet Gynecol.* 2010 Nov;203(5):499.e1-5.

Mereu L, Carri G, Khalifa H. Robotic single port total laparoscopic hysterectomy for endometrial cancer patients. *Gynecol Oncol* 2012; 127:644.

Merlin TL, Hiller JE, Maddern GJ, Jamieson GG, Brown AR, Kolbe A. Systematic review of the safety and effectiveness of methods used to establish pneumoperitoneum in laparoscopic surgery. *Br J Surg* 2003; 90: 668-679.

Mettler L, Nikam YA.A comparative survey of various uterine manipulators used in operative laparoscopy. *Gynecol Surg.* 2006; 3: 239-43.

Moberg AC, Montgomery A. Primary access-related complications with laparoscopy: comparison of blind and open techniques. *Surg Endosc* 2005; 19: 1196-1199.

Moran ME. Rossum's universal robots: not the machines. *J Endourol.* 2007 Dec;21(12):1399-402.

Moran ME. The da Vinci robot. J Endourol. 2006 Dec;20(12):986-90.

Nakib G, Calcaterra V, Scorletti F, Romano P, Goruppi I, Mencherini S, Avolio L, Pelizzo G. Robotic assisted surgery in pediatric gynecology: promising innovation in mini invasive surgical procedures. J Pediatr Adolesc Gynecol. 2013 Feb;26(1):e5-7.

Narducci F1, Collinet P, Merlot B, Lambaudie E, Boulanger L, Lefebvre-Kuntz D, Nickers P, Taieb S, Houvenaeghel G, Leblanc E. Benefit of robot-assisted laparoscopy in nerve-sparing radical hysterectomy: urinary morbidity in early cervical cancer. *Surg Endosc.* 2013 Apr;27(4):1237-42.

Nawfal AK, Eisenstein D, Theoharis E, Dahlman M, Wegienka G. Vaginal cuff closure during robotic-assisted total laparoscopic hysterectomy: comparing vicryl to barbed sutures. *JSLS.* 2012 Oct-Dec;16(4):525-9.

Nezhat C, Hajhosseini B, King LP. Robotic-assisted laparoscopic treatment of bowel, bladder, and ureteral endometriosis. *JSLS.* 2011 Jul-Sep;15(3):387-92.

Nezhat C, Lavie O, Lemyre M, Gemer O, Bhagan L, Nezhat C. Laparoscopic hysterectomy with and without a robot: Stanford experience. *JSLS.* 2009 Apr-Jun;13(2):125-8.

Nezhat C, Lewis M, Kotikela S, Veeraswamy A, Saadat L, Hajhosseini B, Nezhat C. Robotic versus standard laparoscopy for the treatment of endometriosis. *Fertil Steril.* 2010 Dec;94(7):2758-60.

Nezhat FR, Pejovic T, Finger TN, Khalil SS. Role of minimally invasive surgery in ovarian cancer. *J Minim Invasive Gynecol.* 2013 Nov-Dec;20(6):754-65.

Nezhat FR, Pejovic T, Finger TN, Khalil SS. Role of minimally invasive surgery in ovarian cancer. *J Minim Invasive Gynecol.* 2013 Nov-Dec;20(6):754-65.

Nicole N, Rachel C, Michael M, Ross B, Sue G, Allison V, Colleen F. Robotic Assisted, Total Laparoscopic, and Total Abdominal Hysterectomy for Management of Uterine Cancer. *J Cancer Ther.* 2012 Apr;3(2):162-166.

Orady M, Hrynewych A, Nawfal AK, Wegienka G. Comparison of robotic-assisted hysterectomy to other minimally invasive approaches. *JSLS.* 2012 Oct-Dec;16(4):542-8.

Ostrzenski A, Ostrzenska KM. Bladder injury during laparoscopic surgery. *Obstet Gynecol.* 1986;53:175–80.

Ozkan O, Akar ME, Ozkan O, Erdogan O, Hadimioglu N, Yilmaz M, Gunseren F, Cincik M, Pestereli E, Kocak H, Mutlu D, Dinckan A, Gecici O, Bektas G, Suleymanlar G. Preliminary results of the first human uterus transplantation from a multiorgan donor. *Fertil Steril.* 2013 Feb;99(2):470-6.

Painvain E, De Pascale A, Carillo C, et al. Preoperative ultrasonic detection of abdominal wall adhesions in laparoscopic surgery. Gynaecol Endosc 1995; 4: 265

Paramasivam S, Proietto A, Puvaneswary M. Pelvic anatomy and MRI. *Best Pract Res Clin Obstet Gynaecol.* 2006 Feb;20(1):3-22.

Pasic RP, Rizzo JA, Fang H, Ross S, Moore M, Gunnarsson C. Comparing robot-assisted with conventional laparoscopic hysterectomy: impact on cost and clinical outcomes. *J Minim Invasive Gynecol.* 2010;17:730–738.

Pathiraja P, Tozzi R. Advances in gynaecological oncology surgery. *Best PractRes Clin Obstet Gynaecol.* 2013 Jun;27(3):415-20.

Patzkowsky KE, As-Sanie S, Smorgick N, Song AH, Advincula AP. Perioperative outcomes of robotic versus laparoscopic hysterectomy for benign disease. *JSLS.* 2013 Jan-Mar;17(1):100-6.

Payne TN, Dauterive FR. A comparison of total laparoscopic hysterectomy to robotically assisted hysterectomy: surgical outcomes in a community practice. *J Minim Invasive Gynecol.* 2008 May-Jun;15(3):286-91.

Pecorelli S. FIGO Committee on Gynacologic Oncology. Revised FIGO staging for carcinoma of the vulva, cervix, and endometrium. *Int JGynaecol Obstet* 2009;105:103-104.

Phong SVN, Koh LKD. Anaesthesia for robotic-assisted radical prostatectomy: considerations for laparoscopy in the Trendelenburg position. *Anaesth Intensive Care* 2007;35:281-5.

Pitter MC, Gargiulo AR, Bonaventura LM, Lehman JS, Srouji SS. Pregnancy outcomes following robot-assisted myomectomy. *Hum Reprod.* 2013 Jan;28(1):99-108.

Prat J; FIGO Committee on Gynecologic Oncology. Staging classification for cancer of the ovary, fallopian tube, and peritoneum. *Int J Gynaecol Obstet.* 2014 Jan;124(1):1-5.

Pundir J, Pundir V, Walavalkar R, Omanwa K, Lancaster G, Kayani S. Robotic-assisted laparoscopic vs abdominal and laparoscopic myomectomy: systematic review and meta-analysis. *J Minim InvasiveGynecol.* 2013 May-Jun;20(3):335-45.

Puntambekar SP, Patil A, Joshi SN, Rayate NV, Puntambekar SS, Agarwal GA. Preservation of autonomic nerves in laparoscopic total radical hysterectomy. *J Laparoendosc Adv Surg Tech A.* 2010 Dec;20(10):813-9.

Quemener J, Boulanger L, Rubod C, Cosson M, Vinatier D, Collinet P. The place of robotics in gynecologic surgery. *J Visc Surg*. 2012 Oct;149(5):e289-301.

Quint EH, Wang FL, Hurd WW. Laparoscopic transillumination for the location of anterior abdominal wall blood vessels. *J Laparoendosc Surg* 1996; 6;167-9.

Ramirez PT, Schmeler KM, Malpica A, Soliman PT. Safety and feasibility of robotic radical trachelectomy in patients with early-stage cervical cancer. *Gynecol Oncol*. 2010 Mar;116(3):512-5.

Rané A, Eng MK, Keeley FX Jr. Port site metastases. *Curr Opin Urol*. 2008 Mar;18(2):185-9.

Reynisson P, Persson J. Hospital costs for robot-assisted laparoscopic radical hysterectomy and pelvic lymphadenectomy. *Gynecol Oncol* 2013;130:95-9.

Robinson BL, Parnell BA, Sandbulte JT, Geller EJ, Connolly A, Matthews CA. Robotic versus vaginal urogynecologic surgery: a retrospective cohort study of perioperative complications in elderly women. Female *Pelvic Med Reconstr Surg*. 2013 Jul-Aug;19(4):230-7.

Robots in Ancient China. Website: http://history.cultural-china.com/en/ 183History4025.html (Accessed: 22/03/2014).

Rodgers AK, Goldberg JM, Hammel JP, Falcone T. Tubal anastomosis by robotic compared with outpatient minilaparotomy. *Obstet Gynecol*. 2007 Jun;109(6):1375-80.

Ross JW, Preston MR. Update on laparoscopic, robotic, and minimally invasive vaginal surgery for pelvic floor repair. *Minerva Ginecol*. 2009 Jun;61(3):173-86.

Rossi EC, Ivanova A, Boggess JF. Robotically assisted fluorescence-guided lymph node mapping with ICG for gynecologic malignancies: a feasibility study. *Gynecol Oncol*. 2012 Jan;124(1):78-82.

Rossi EC, Jackson A, Ivanova A, Boggess JF. Detection of sentinel nodes for endometrial cancer with robotic assisted fluorescence imaging: cervical versus hysteroscopic injection. *Int J Gynecol Cancer*. 2013 Nov;23(9):1704-11.

Saceanu S, Cela V, Surlin V, Angelescu CM, Patrascu S, Georgescu I, Genazzani A. Hysterectomy for benign uterine pathology: comparison between robotic assisted laparoscopy, classic laparoscopy and laparotomy. *Chirurgia* (Bucur). 2013 May-Jun;108(3):346-50.

Salicrú SR, de la Torre JF, Gil-Moreno A. The surgical management of early-stage cervical cancer. *Curr Opin Obstet Gynecol*. 2013 Aug;25(4):312-9.

Sánchez Martín FM, Millán Rodríguez F, Salvador Bayarri J, Palou Redorta J, Rodríguez Escovar F, Esquena Fernández S, Villavicencio Mavrich H. [History of robotics: from Archytas of Tarentum until da Vinci robot. (Part I)]. *Actas Urol Esp*. 2007;31(2):69-76.

Sarlos D, Kots L, Stevanovic N, Schaer G. Robotic hysterectomy versus conventional laparoscopic hysterectomy: outcome and cost analyses of a matched case-control study. *Eur J Obstet Gynecol Reprod Biol*. 2010 May;150(1):92-6.

Schreuder HW, Verheijen RH. Robotic surgery. *BJOG*. 2009 Jan;116(2):198-213.

Seamon LG, Cohn DE, Richardson DL, Hurt JD, Nickerson EC, Fowler JM. Robotic pelvic and aortic lymphadenectomy for endometrial cancer: the console surgeon's perspectives on surgical technique and directing the assistant. *J Minim Invasive Gynecol*. 2010 Mar-Apr;17(2):180-5.

Seamon LG, Fowler JM, Richardson DL, Carlson MJ, Valmadre S, Phillips GS, Cohn DE. A detailed analysis of the learning curve: robotic hysterectomy and pelvic-aortic lymphadenectomy for endometrial cancer. *Gynecol Oncol.* 2009 Aug;114(2):162-7.

Sert MB, Eraker R. Robot-assisted laparoscopic surgery in gynaecological oncology; initial experience at Oslo Radium Hospital and 16 months follow-up. *Int J Med Robot.* 2009 Dec;5(4):410-4.

Sgarbura O, Vasilescu C. The decisive role of the patient-side surgeon in robotic surgery. *Surg Endosc.* 2010 Dec;24(12):3149-55.

Shah NT, Wright KN, Jonsdottir GM, Jorgensen S, Einarsson JI, Muto MG. The Feasibility of Societal Cost Equivalence between Robotic Hysterectomy and Alternate Hysterectomy Methods for Endometrial Cancer. *Obstet Gynecol Int* 2011;2011:570464.

Shashoua AR, Gill D, Locher SR. Robotic-assisted total laparoscopic hysterectomy versus conventional total laparoscopic hysterectomy. *JSLS.* 2009 Jul-Sep;13(3):364-9.

Smith AL, Scott EM, Krivak TC, Olawaiye AB, Chu T, Richard SD. Dual-console robotic surgery: a new teaching paradigm. *J Robot Surg.* 2013 Jun;7(2):113-118.

Smith JA, Jr., Herrell SD. Robotic-assisted laparoscopic prostatectomy: do minimally invasive approaches offer significant advantages? J Clin Oncol 2005;23:8170-5.

Soderstrom RM. Injuries to major blood vessels during endoscopy. *J AmAssoc Gynecol Laparosc* 1997; 4: 395-8.

Soto E, Lo Y, Friedman K, Soto C, Nezhat F, Chuang L, Gretz H Total laparoscopic hysterectomy versus da Vinci robotic hysterectomy: is using the robot beneficial? *J Gynecol Oncol.* 2011 Dec;22(4):253-9.

Sur RL, Wagner AA, Albala DM, Su LM. Critical role of the assistant in laparoscopic and robot-assisted radical prostatectomy. *J Endourol.* 2008 Apr;22(4):587-9; discussion 589-90.

Tarnay CM, Glass KB, Munro MG. Incision characteristics associated with six laparoscopic trocar-cannula systems: a randomized, observer-blinded comparison. *Obstet Gynecol* 1999; 94: 89-93.

Teoh B, Sen R, Abbott J. An evaluation of four tests used to ascertain Veres needle placement at closed laparoscopy. *J Minim Invasive Gynecol.* 2005;12:153–8.

Thiel DD, Lannen A, Richie E, Dove J, Gajarawala NM, Igel TC. Simulation-based training for bedside assistants can benefit experienced robotic prostatectomy teams. *J Endourol.* 2013 Feb;27(2):230-7.

Ulmer BC. Best practices for minimally invasive procedures. *AORN J.* 2010 May;91(5):558-72.

Uppal S, Frumovitz M, Escobar P, Ramirez PT. Laparoendoscopic single-site surgery in gynecology: review of literature and available technology. *J Minim Invasive Gynecol* 2011; 18:12–23.

van Dam P, Hauspy J, Verkinderen L, et al. Are costs of robot-assisted surgery warranted for gynecological procedures? *Obstet Gynecol Int* 2011;2011:973830.

Verheijen R, Zweemer R. Robotic surgery for gynaecologic cancer: an overview. *Curr Oncol Rep.* 2012 Dec;14(6):544-9.

Vick CW, WalshJW, WheelockJB, Brewer WH. CT of the normal and abnormal parametria in cervical cancer. *AJR* 1984; 143:597-603.

Visco AG, Advincula AP. Robotic gynecologic surgery. *Obstet Gynecol.* 2008 Dec;112(6):1369-84.

Vitobello D, Siesto G, Bulletti C, Accardi A, Iedà N. Robotic radical parametrectomy with pelvic lymphadenectomy: our experience and review of the literature. *Eur J Surg Oncol.* 2012 Jun;38(6):548-54.

Weber DM. Laparoscopic surgery: an excellent approach in elderly patients. *Arch Surg.* 2003 Oct;138(10):1083-8.

Weber ED, Colyer MH, Lesser RL, Subramanian PS. Posterior ischemic optic neuropathy after minimally invasive prostatectomy. *J Neuroophthalmol.* 2007 Dec;27(4):285-7.

Weinberg L, Rao S, Escobar PF. Robotic surgery in gynecology: an updated systematic review. *Obstet Gynecol Int.* 2011;2011:852061.

Yates DR, Vaessen C, Roupret M. From Leonardo to da Vinci: the history of robot-assisted surgery in urology. *BJU Int.* 2011;108(11):1708-13.

Yim GW, Kim SW, Nam EJ, Kim YT. Role of robot-assisted surgery in cervical cancer. *Int J Gynecol Cancer.* 2011 Jan;21(1):173-81.

Yim GW, Kim YT. Robotic surgery in gynecologic cancer. *Curr Opin ObstetGynecol.* 2012 Feb;24(1):14-23.

Yuh B. The bedside assistant in robotic surgery--keys to success. *Urol Nurs.* 2013 Jan-Feb;33(1):29-32.

Zakashansky K, Bradley WH, Chuang L, Rahaman J, Dottino P. Recent advances in the surgical management of cervical cancer. *Mt Sinai J Med.* 2009 Dec;76(6):567-76.

Index

E

F

G

H

I

K

L

M

N

O

P

Q

R

S

U

V

W

X